Handbook For Microbiology Practice In Oral And Maxillofacial Diagnosis

A study guide to laboratory
techniques in Oral Microbiology

Arvind Babu RS, BDS., MDS., DFO.,
Oral and Maxillofacial Pathologist,
Lecturer and Research Coordinator,
Dentistry Programme, Faculty of Medical Sciences,
The University of the West Indies,
Mona, Kingston 7,
Jamaica, West Indies.

Reddy BVR, BDS., MDS.,
Prof and Head,
Dept of Oral and Maxillofacial
Pathology and Microbiology,
SIBAR Institute of Dental Sciences,
Takkellapadu, Guntur,
Andhra Pradesh.

Chandrasekar P, BDS., MDS.,
Reader,
Dept. of Oral and Maxillofacial
Pathology and Microbiology,
SIBAR Institute of Dental Sciences,
Takkellapadu, Guntur,
Andhra Pradesh.

Anuradha CH, BDS., MDS.,
Reader,
Dept. of Oral and Maxillofacial
Pathology and Microbiology,
Sree Sai Dental College and
Research Institute,
Chapuram, Srikakulam,
Andhra Pradesh, India.

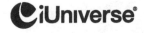

HANDBOOK FOR MICROBIOLOGY PRACTICE IN ORAL AND MAXILLOFACIAL DIAGNOSIS
A STUDY GUIDE TO LABORATORY TECHNIQUES IN ORAL MICROBIOLOGY

iUniverse books may be ordered through booksellers or by contacting:

iUniverse LLC
1663 Liberty Drive
Bloomington, IN 47403
www.iuniverse.com
1-800-Authors (1-800-288-4677)

Because of the dynamic nature of the Internet, any web addresses or links contained in this book may have changed since publication and may no longer be valid. The views expressed in this work are solely those of the author and do not necessarily reflect the views of the publisher, and the publisher hereby disclaims any responsibility for them.

Any people depicted in stock imagery provided by Thinkstock are models, and such images are being used for illustrative purposes only.
Certain stock imagery © Thinkstock.

ISBN: 978-1-4917-2869-7 (sc)
ISBN: 978-1-4917-2870-3 (e)

Library of Congress Control Number: 2014905633

Print information available on the last page.

iUniverse rev. date: 7/27/2015

CONTENTS

Contents

This work is dedicated to the noblest profession of
Dentistry and Oral Pathology and Microbiology,
Patients, in whose absence; we would never understand
the cause and nature of disease and teachers,
beloved parents, wife, colleagues and seniors.

PREFACE

Oral Microbiology is a study of microbial diseases of oral cavity. For the depth and precision of knowledge to this noble field, it can be divided in to clinical and practical aspects of microbiology. Oral microbiology denotes the congregation of basic medical sciences and practising dentistry. The most common oral microbial disease and present ever since olden days of earth is dental caries. Also, there are many microbiological diseases that affect the oral cavity. Often there are diverse list of microbes that can target the oral tissues. These microbial diseases can cause potential tissue damage; or majority of time it leads to compromised oral health; also some times it can escort to death. There is available number of literatures over the microbial diseases. But, the state of morbidity and mortality factors associated with these microbial diseases leaves an important and special enlightenment of oral microbiology in terms of diagnostic procedures are needed. Since it has no technique of its own, comprehension of this special field has to be drawn and adapted from the disciplines of medical microbiology. The context of bringing this book is an attempt to get an attention towards diagnostic procedure and laboratory techniques that are emphasized over the oral microbiological practice. This text book tried an initial attempt to bring the practical knowledge microbiological techniques in the context of dental diagnostician. Besides, if there are any errors in the textual content, it is advised to reader to bring it to authors notice to make the corrections in the future editions.

Dr. Arvind Babu RS., B.D.S., M.D.S., D.F.O.,
Oral and Maxillofacial Pathologist and Microbiologist
Lecturer and Research Coordinator,
Faculty of Medical Sciences—Dentistry Programme,
The University of West Indies, Mona campus,
Kingston—7, Jamaica.

1

INTRODUCTION

Medical Microbiology:

Study of microbes that infects humans, the disease they cause, their diagnosis, prevention and treatment. It also deals with response of human, host to microbial and other antigens.

Varo and Columella (1st Century) suggested that disease caused by invisible beings called animal minuta, which is from the inhaled / ingested particles.

Fra castorius of Verona 1546, suggested that contagium vivum caused the possible infection.

Von ptenciz 1762, suggested each disease was caused by separate agents.

Kircher 1659, reported minute worms in blood of plague victims.

Antony von Leuwenhoek first observed and reported the

bacteria. He is a draper (Clothing) in delft Holland, he had hobby of grinding lenses and observed some diverse materials through them. He made accurate description of various types of bacteria and communicated to ROYAL SOCIETY of LONDON.

Leuwenhoek termed the world of little animal cules.

Later 2 centuries the importance of animal cules came in medicine and biology as a whole came to be recognized.

Augustino Bassi 1835, showed the fungus in muscardine disease of silkworms.

Davaome and Pollander 1850, observed anthrx bacilli in the blood of animals dying in disease.

Oliver Wendell holmes (1843) suggested that puerpal contagious.

Semmel wein identified mode of transmission by doctors and medical students, attending women in labour in hospital and he had prevented it by the simple measure of wasting hands in antiseptic solutions.

Louis Pasteur in 1822-95, studied on fermentation, also suggested different types of fermentation with different micro organisms.

Needham Irish priest 1745, contradicted Louis pastuer, and suggested that microbes generation by putrescible fluid.

Pasteur introduced techniques of sterilization and developed steam sterilizer, hot air oven and auto clave.

Pasteur started studies on pebrine, anthrax, chicken pox, cholera and Hydrophobia.

—An accidental finding that chicken cholera bacillus cultures left on bench for several weeks lost their pathogenic property, but retained their ability to protect the birds against subsequent infection by attenuation.

—He attenuated cultures of anthrax bacillus by incubation at high temperature 42-43°C and proved this gives specific protection against anthrax.

—Pasteur coined the term vaccine, for his first preparation for cow pox.

Lister 1867, step from Pasteur work, introduced aspectic technique in surgery, and there was drop in mortality and morbidity due to surgical sepsis.

He used carbolic acid, actually cumber some and hazardous. It was milestone in evolution of surgical practice from the era of laudable pus to modern septic technique.

PASTEUR LAID FOUNDATION OF MICROBIOLOGY.

Robert Koch 1843-1910.

Cultured and studied life cycle of anthrax.

Introduced staining technique and methods of obtaining bacteria in pure culture using solid media.

Discovered the bacillus of tuberculosis (1882) and cholera Vibrio.

Hansen 1874—leprosy bacillus.

Niesser 1879—gonococcus.

Ogsion 1881—staphylococcus.

Loeffler 1884—diphtheria bacillus

Nicoler 1884—tetanus bacilli.

Frankel 1886—pneumococcus.

Schauddin and Hoffman 1905—syphilis.

Roux and yersin : mechanism of pathogens in diphtheria by toxin and suggested toxins neutralized by anti toxins.

Ehrlich studied toxins and Antitoxins laid foundation for biological standarisation.

Like wise slowly, causative agents of various different disease was reported by different investigation, it was necessary to introduce criteria for proving and Claim that microorganism in pathogenicity.

These criteria was actually introduced by Henle, and enunciated by Koch called as Koch's postulates:

1. Bacterium should be constantly associated with the lesion of disease.
2. It should be possible to isolate the bacterium in pure culture fro the lesion.
3. Inoculation of such pure culture in to suitable laboratory animals should reproduce the lesions of disease.
4. It should be possible to re—isolate the bacterium in the pure culture from lesion produced in experimental animals.
5. **AN ADDITIONAL CRITERIA:**
   Specific antibodies to the bacterium should be demonstrable in the serum of patients suffereing from the disease.
   It is not always be positive to satisfy all the postulates, extremely useful in doubts regarding the causative agents.

By 20th century many infectious disease had been proved to be caused by bacteria.

But, there remained a large No. of disease like Small pox, chicken pox, measles, influenza and common cold for which no bacterial cause could be made.

Pasteur, during his investigation of rabies in dogs, Pasteur suspected that disease could be caused by a microbe too small to be seen even under a microscope.

Ivanosky 1892, suggested existence of such ultra microscopic microbes.

Beijernick 1898, coined the term virus.

Loeffler and frosch 1898, hand foot mouth disease of cattle caused by small filter passing virus.

Ist viral disease in Human was yellow fever, transmitted by infected microbes.

Virus was difficult to visualize in light microscope, as it couldnot be seen.

Introduction of Electron microscope and Ruska in 1934 refinement in electron microscopic techniques, made to visualize virus.

Cultivation of virus was possible only in animals / human volunteer till technique of growing them on chick embryo developed by good Pasteur in 1930.

Virus could lead to malignancy was put by ellerman and Bang in 1908.

Peyton rous in 1911, isolated a virus causing sarcoma in fowls.

Discovery of virus and cellular oncogenes has shed light on the possible mechanism of viral oncogenesis.

It is noticed that persons surviving from the attack of small pox did not develop the disease when exposed to the infection for second time.

This led to an idea of prevention of disease by producing mild form of small pox virus intentionally called as variolation.

It was observed that immunity to small pox in milk maid who were exposed to occupational cow pox infection, introduced the technique of vaccination using cow pox material 1796.

Pasteur given vaccine against cholera, anthrax and rabies.

Von behria and Kitasato suggested the antibody and humoral factor in immunology.

Prior experience with microorganism / other antigen did not always result in beneficial effect or immunity / protection. At times it caused opposite effect.

Koch in 1890, noticed when the tubercle bacillus or its protein was injected in to a guinea pig already infected with the bacillus an exaggerated response takes place called hypersensitivity reaction.

Richet 1902, studying the toxic extracts of seas anemones in dog, make the paradoxical observation that dogs had prior contact with toxin were abnormal sensitive to even minute, termed as anaphylaxis. This developed the phenomenon of allergy, characteristic feature of immunity, whether protective / destructive (allergy).

Explaination for exquisite specificity of immunological reaction had to await the advances in protein chemistry.

Landsteiner laid the foundation of immunochemistry. Chemist dominated the study of immunity for several decades and theories of antibody synthesis were postulated by them.

Immunological process in health and disease are now better understood following the identification of two components of immunity

1. Humoral (antibody mediated)
2. Cellular immunity (cell mediated—T cell)

Thomas in 1959, Burnet in 1967, developed the concept of immunological survillence.

Primary function of immune system is to pressure integrity of body, seeking and destroying all foreign antigens, autogenous external in origin.

Malignancy was visualized as a failure of this function and the scope of immunity was enlarged to include the natural defense against cancer.

Understanding the immunological basis of transplantation, role of immunity in rejection of transplantation made to find MHC / HLA by medawaar and Burnet. Who made successful transplants.

Blood transfusion—Landsteiner 1900 who did the blood grouping.

Accidental discovery that fungus pencillium produces a substances which destroy the staphylococcus, second world war was beginning of antibiotic era.

Rapidly so many antibiotics was discovered hoped that bacterial infection would be controlled with in a short period, but soon development of drug resistance in bacteria presented serious difficulties.

Discovery of antibiotics, vaccine against bacterial and viral disease raised the expectations and eventual elimination of all infectious disease.

Global eradication of small pox inspired vision of world.

But invariably, new infections started began to appear, 1981 when AIDS was identified in USA, and Pandemic spread it was realized that controlling microbes is a most difficult task than it was imagined.

As part fro benefits like methods of diagnosis, prevention, treatment, control of infectious disease, medical microbiology contributed to scientific knowledge in many ways.

1. Unraveling genetic code.
2. Molecular level mysteries in biology.
3. Recombinant DNA technology.
4. Genetic and molecular emergency.

2

CLASSIFICATION OF MICROBES

1. **Classification based on the fundamental structure on microbial organism cell.**

UNICELLULAR ORGANISMS
(Classified in descending order of complexity as)

Eukaryotes
Protozoa and Fungi
Rickettsiae

Prokaryotes
bacteria, Mycoplasmas,

and chlamydiae.

2. **Classification based on pathogenic organism**

MICROBES

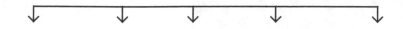

BACTERIA FUNGI VIRUS PROTOZOA PARASITES

3. <u>Classification of bacteria based on their shapes</u>

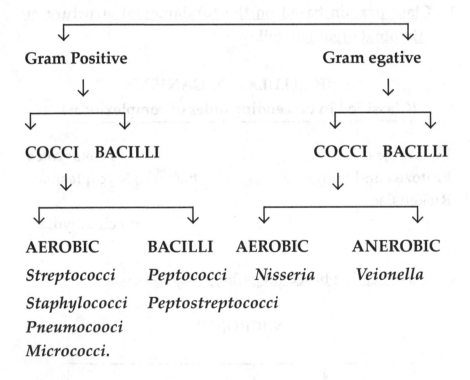

BACTERIA

COCCI BACILLI VIBRIO SPIRELLA SPIROCHAETE

4. <u>Classification of bacteria—based on gram staining and aerobic / anaerobic nature:</u>

BACTERIA

Gram Positive   Gram egative

COCCI BACILLI   COCCI BACILLI

AEROBIC	BACILLI	AEROBIC	ANEROBIC
Streptococci	*Peptococci*	*Nisseria*	*Veionella*
Staphylococci	*Peptostreptococci*		
Pneumocooci			
Micrococci.			

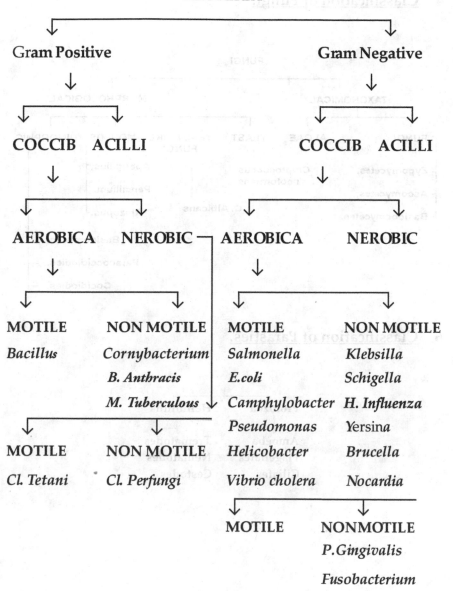

4. <u>Classification of Fungi:</u>

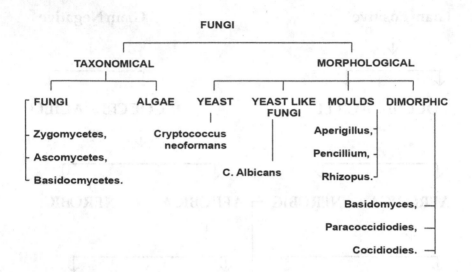

6. <u>Classification of Parasties.</u>

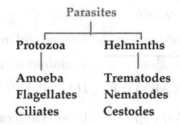

7. Classification of Viurs based on genomic content:

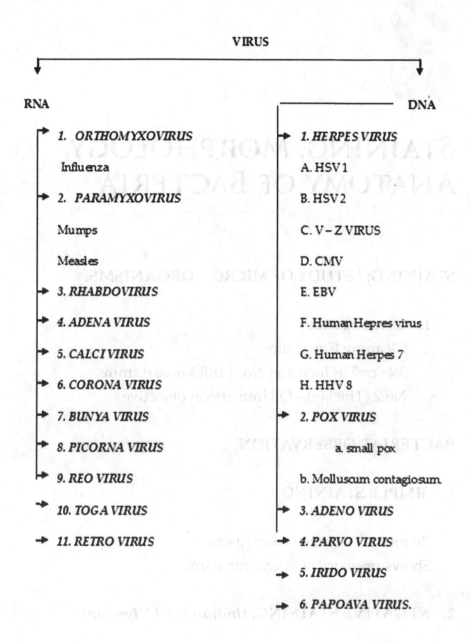

VIRUS

RNA

1. *ORTHOMYXOVIRUS*

Influenza

2. *PARAMYXOVIRUS*

Mumps

Measles

3. *RHABDOVIRUS*

4. *ADENA VIRUS*

5. *CALCI VIRUS*

6. *CORONA VIRUS*

7. *BUNYA VIRUS*

8. *PICORNA VIRUS*

9. *REO VIRUS*

10. *TOGA VIRUS*

11. *RETRO VIRUS*

DNA

1. *HERPES VIRUS*

A. HSV 1

B. HSV 2

C. V – Z VIRUS

D. CMV

E. EBV

F. Human Hepres virus

G. Human Herpes 7

H. HHV 8

2. *POX VIRUS*

a. small pox

b. Molluscum contagiosum

3. *ADENO VIRUS*

4. *PARVO VIRUS*

5. *IRIDO VIRUS*

6. *PAPOAVA VIRUS.*

3

Staining, Morphology, Anatomy of Bacteria

STAINING: / STUDY OF MICRO—ORGANISMS.

1. Cleaning slide
2. Cleaning Cover slips.
   3/4th or 7/8th inch and No. 1 thickness 0.1mm
   No.2 (Thicker)—Oil immersion objective

BACTERIAL OBSERVATION

1. SIMPLE STAINING

By methylene blue / basic fuschin.
Shows presence of microorganism.

2. NEGATIVE STAINING: *(Indian ink / Nigrosin)*

Provide uniform colored background against which unstained bacteria is seen. Bacteria size, shape can be seen.

10% Nigrosin is made in warm distill water.

Add formalin 0.5%

Small drop of dye placed over slide.

Examining fluid mixed with dye.

Spread dye and Fluid.

3. Impregnation method:

Bacterial cell is too thin to view in microscope, Impregnation of silver on surface.

Used for demonstration of spirocheate and bacterial flagella.

4. Differential staining:

Stains impart different colors to different bacteria / structure of bacteria (cell wall)

Gram staining (Table 1 shows the conventional method and Table 2 shows the modification in gram staining methods)

Acid fast staining.

Table 1: GRAM STAINING—Preston— morell modified gram staining method

COMPONENTS OF GRAM STAINING:	DYES
1. PRIMARY DYE (1 minute)	Para Rosanilne dyes—Methyl violet / crystal violet / Gentian violet. (basic dye)
2. FIXATIVE / MORDANT. (1 minute)	Gram's Iodine
3. DECOLORIZER. (10-30 seconds)	Alcohol / Acetone
4. COUNTER STAIN (30 seconds)	Safarin / dilute carbol fuschin / neutral red

GRAM POSITIVE	GRAM NEGATIVE
Resist decolorization and retain primary stain appears violet / dark violet	Decolorised by organic solution (Acetone) Take up counter stain, appear pink / red

COMMON ERRORS IN STAINING PROCEDURE

1. Excessive heat during fixation
2. Low concentration of crystal violet
3. Excessive washing between steps
4. Insufficient iodine exposure
5. Prolonged decolourization
6. Excessive counterstaining

Artefacts in Gram Staining

1. Gram stain reagents (Crystal Violet, Iodine, Safranin and Neutral Red
2. Dirty glass slides
3. Contaminated water used to rinse slides

MECHANISM OF GRAM STAINING

1. **PERMEABILITY OF CELL WALL and CYTOPLASMIC MEMBRANE:**

   1. Gram +ve cells have more acidic protoplasm, which accounts for retaining basic dye.
   2. Iodine makes the protoplasm more acidic and serves mordant.
   3. Gram +ve cell wall less permeable, dye—iodine complex traped in cell resist outflow by decoloriser.
   4. Gm—ve organism : increased premeable to acetone, hence outflow of dye iodine complex.

2. **Integrity of cell wall:**

   Integrity of cell wall is essential.

   Gram positive organism becomes gram negative if the cell wall is damaged.

Table 2: MODIFICATION OF GRAM STAINING

METHOD	MODIFICATION
Kopeleff and beerman's modification	Acetone as decoloriser
Jensen's Modification	Alcohol as decoloriser
Weiger's modification	Aniline xylol as decoloriser
Preston's and Morell modification	Iodine acetone as decoloriser.
Modified preston—Morell gram staining method	Weak—iodine acetone is used because it's a irritant aerosol.

Acetone as decoloriser appears to give more specific reactions than alcohol. But it acts so quickly. Addition of small concentration of iodine to acetone slow down the rate of decolorisation without reducing its specificity.

ACID FAST STAINING

- It's differential staining of tubercle bacilli and other acid fast bacilli with Aniline gentian violet followed by strong nitric acid.
- *Mycobacterium / certain bacterium are difficult to stain and once stain, it resist decolorisation.—hence acid fast stain.*
- The components of Acid fast staining method and action of the same are shown in table 3.

Table 3: Composition of Acid fast staining

CONTENTS	ACTION
Carbol Fuschin	Basic dye.
20% sulphuric acid	Decolorize.
2% methylene blue	Counter stain.

PROCEDURE:

1. Heat is applied to undersurface of slide, by flame untill stain steams.
2. Carbol fuschin stain poured on a slide containing smear. (5-10 mts.)
3. Wash with water.
4. Decolorise—20% H2so4.
5. Counter stain with—2% methylene blue—for 1-2 minutes.
6. Wash with water.
7. Acid fast bacilli—retain duschin red color.

4

Ph Measurements, Buffer, Oxidation— Reduction Potential.

1. pH: Logarthimic reciprocal value of H ion concentration.
2. Micro—organisms are susceptible to change the acidity / alkalinity of surrounding medium. pH is important for growth and their survival.
3. Bacteria grow widely ranging from acidic to alkaline.
a. 2 types of method employed for pH measurement. (Table 4) pH meter. pH indicator dyes.
4. Indicators and their range of pH with color categorization (Table 5)
5. "Organisms are sensitive to changes in acidity because H+ and OH-interfere with H bonding in proteins and nucleic acids"

Table 4: pH meter and pH dyes

pH meter	pH dyes
Accurate method to measure pH	Substances that will change in color with variations in the pH of solutions.
Consists—pair of electrodes, sensitive to H + ions. (Principle: Measures Electro—motive forces EMF)	Eg: Phenol sulphone—pthalein It is yellow in acid solution, red in alkaline solution.

Table 5 Indicators and their range of pH with color categorization

INDICATOR	RANGE of pH	COLOR CHANGE
Thymol blue (acid range)	1.2-2.8	Red to yellow
Bromophenol blue	2.8-4.6	Yellow to violet.
Bromocresol green	3.6-5.2	Yellow to blue
Methyl red	4.4-6.2	Red to yellow
Litmus	4.5-8.3	Red to blue
Bromocresol purple	5.2-6.8	Yellow to violet
Bromocresol blue	6.0-7.6	Yellow to blue
Neutral red	6.8-8.0	Red to yellow
Phenol red	6.8-8.4	Yellow to purple pink
Cresol red	7.2-8.8	Yellow to violet red
Thymol blue	8.0-9.6	Yellow to blue
Phenolphthalein	8.3-10.0	Colorless to red

Thymolpththalein	9.3-10.5	Colorless to blue
BDH (Universal)	3.011.0	Red orange— yellow—green blue—blue— reddish violet

BUFFERS

1. Micro—organisms produce acids / alkali as a result of metabolic activities and these must be prevented from altering the pH of environment.

2. Eg: bacteria when grown on a medium containing a sugar generally produce acid intermediates or end products (formic acid, acetic acid, propionic acid or lactic acid). This is particularly true of fermentation under relatively anaerobic conditions.

3. If these acidic products were allowed to accumulate in an unbuffered medium, the organism would soon be killed by low pH produced.

4. Buffers are formed from mixing weak acid with its acid. (Table 6)

   Eg: 0.1 mol / Lt of Acetic acid dissoved in 0.1 mol / Lt of Sodium acetate

5. BUFFER'S TEND TO RESIST CHANGES IN H+ ION CONCENTRATION.

Table 6: Buffer and salt

BUFFER	WEAK ACID	SALT
Citrate buffer	Citric acid	Sodium citrate
Acetate buffer	Acetic acid	Sodium acetate
Citrate— phosphate buffer	Citric acid	Di basic sodium phosphate
Phosphate buffer	Monobasic sodium phosphate	Dibasic sodium phosphate
Barbitone (veronal)	Sodium barbitone	HCl
Tris (Hydroxy methyl) amino methane HCl (Tris Hcl buffer)	Tris (hydroxy methyl) Aminomethane	HCl
Boric acid—Borax buffer	Boric acid	Borax
Carbonate— bicarbonate buffer	Anhydrous sodium carbonate	Sodium Bicarbonate

Oxidation—reduction potential

1. Strict aerobes grow in presence of O2.
2. Strict anaerobes require Reducing condition.
3. Anaerobes cannot grow in Oxygenated environment due to production of H202, which cannot be removed by catalases.
4. This relates to the metabolic character of the organism and helps to grow in culture in media and species identification.

REDOX

1. Oxidising substance capable of taking up electrons.
2. Reducing agents—capable to part with electrons.
3. Net ability of readiness of all component is expressed by REDOX potential.
4. Redox potential measured by electrode immersed in a solution. (Table 7)

Electrode potential (Eh) :

More in oxidised system (Higher / Positive potential)

Less in Reduced system (Lower / Negative potential)

Platinum electrode

Redox potential are measured by electrical method, also special dyes can be used—color indicator of redox potentials.

Table 7: Showing Redox dye and it's potential at pH 7.0

Redox dye	Redox potential at pH7.0
Methylene blue	+11 mv
Resazurin	-42 mv
Phenosaffarine	-252 mv
Neutral dye	-325 mv

5

CULTURE MEDIA

A *Culture medium* is nothing but the nutrients, prepared and supplied for artificial growth of microorganisms. A *Sterilere culture medium* is one which does not have any living microbes. *Inoculum* is nothing but the introduction of microbes into medium. A *Culture* represents the Microbes growing in /on culture medium.

Different organisms have widely differing nutritional requirements. Hence, it must be ensured that the culture medium used in the laboratory meets the needs of the organism to be cultured.

Criteria To Be Observed:

We should ensure that the source of carbon, energy and nitrogen is given in the form of amino acids and carbohydrates. Characters of a good culture medium are—

1. It should possess Nutrients, Ions and Moisture, in the correct proportions.
2. It should have a Correct pH and osmotic pressure.

3. It should be able to Neutralize any toxic material produced.

4. It is essential to incubate in the correct atmosphere (aerobic / anaerobic) and optimum temperature, for adequate period.

Culture Media

(Based on Ingredients)

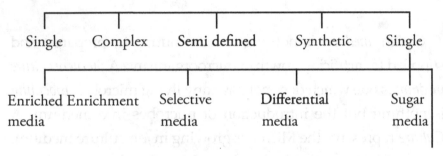

CLASSIFICATION OF CULTURE MEDIA:

1. CLASSIFICATION BASED ON INGREDIENTS:

1. Simple Media
2. Complex Media
3. Synthetic or defined media
4. Semi defined Media
5. Special Media—They are again of the following types—

   i. Enriched Media
   ii. Selective—incl. Enrichment Media
   iii. Indicator / Differential Media

2. Identification Media, based on the biochemical reactions

   1. Transport Media
   2. Storage Media

3. CLASSIFICATION BASED ON THE CONSITENCY OF MEDIA:

   1. Solid media
   2. Liquid media
   3. Semisolid media

4. CLASSIFICATION BASED ON THE ATMOSPHERE OF OXYGEN:

   1. Aerobic media
   2. Anaerobic media

5. CLASSIFICATION BASED ON THE ORGANISM ISOLATED:

   1. Bacterial culture media
   2. Fungal culture media
   3. Parasitic culture media

PURPOSE OF CULTURE MEDIA:

1. Chemically defined culture media: Growth of chemoautotrophs and photoautotrophs and microbiological assays.

2. Comple media : Growth of most chemoheterotrophic organisms.
3. Reducing media : Growth of obligate anaerobes.
4. Selective media: suppression of unwanted microbes; encouraging desired microbes.
5. Differential media : Differentiation of colonies of desired microbes from others.
6. Enrichment media: Similar to selective media but designed to increase numbers of desired microbes to detectable levels.

TYPES OF CULTURE MEDIA:

1. **SYNTETIC (Defined) MEDIA:** They are prepared by adding precise amounts of highly purified inorganic or organic chemicals to distilled water. So, the exact chemical composition of medium is known.
2. **COMPLEX MEDIA:** These media are prepared by adding digests of casein (milk protein), beef, soybeans, yeast cells and other highly nutritious but chemically undefined substances.
3. **NUTRIENT MEDIA:** These are the simple complex media, containing peptone and agar.

SPECIAL GROWTH MEDIA:

1. **ENRICHED MEDIA:** These are the nutrient media containing enrichments such as blood or serum or yeast extract. Enrichment provides additional growth

factors for more fastidious organisms (includes many pathogens). e.g. Blood agar.

2. **ENRICHMENT MEDIA:** The Enrichment media are those which contain special nutrients that allow the growth of a particular organism that may be present in low numbers and so masked by other organisms. They are usually in the form of a broth culture medium. e.g. Rappaport's medium for Salmonella; Enterococcosal Broth for Enterococci.

3. **SELECTIVE MEDIA:** The selective medium encourages the growth of some organisms but suppresses the growth of others. e.g. Mannitol salt agar for isolation of *Staphylococcus aureus.*

4. **DIFFERENTIAL MEDIA:** They have a constituent that causes an observable change (change in colour or change in pH) in the medium when a particular biochemical reaction occurs. e.g. Fermentation of lactose in MacConkey medium causes a pH change, which enables the Lactose fermenting colonies to appear pink, and non-lactose-fermenting colonies to be colourless.

5. **COMBINED SELECTIVE and DIFFERENTIAL MEDIA:** These media have the properties of both Selective and also the differential media. e.g. MacConkey Agar containing crystal violet and bile salts (inhibit Gram-positive bacteria) + Lactose + pH indicator.

COMPONENTS OF MEDIA:

The media which are used for culturing the organisms should contain the following

a. General nutrient sources like Peptones, and water soluble protein hydrolysates which are in the form of infusions (extracts)
b. Specific growth factors (vitamins, amino acids) pH indicators
c. Reducing agents and
d. Selective agents

Pure Cultures: A pure culture contains only one species or strain. A colony is a population of cells arising from a single cell or spore or from a group of attached cells. A colony is often called a colony-forming unit (CFU).

AGAR-AGAR: Agar-Agar is a complex polysaccharide which is extracted from seaweeds. It is used as a solidifying agent for preparing solid culture media in Petri plates, slants, and in deeps. It is usually available as a purified and dried up powder. It is generally not metabolized by microbes. It contains the following—

- Long chain polysaccharide D-Galatopyranose units.
- Mg and Ca sulphates.

The physical properties of Agar are—

- It is non nutritive and does not alter the pH.

- It liquefies at 100°C.
- It Solidifies at 40°C.
- To obtain the Solid media, 1-2% agar is essential for hardening.
- Whereas in the Semisolid media, 0.2-0.4% of agar is essential.
- Jellifying property of the New Zealand agar is more than that of the Japanese Agar.

PEPTONE:

It is usually obtained from the Lean meat heart muscle, casein, fibrin, soya flour, pepsin, trypsin, and papain. It contains Peptones, Proteones, Amino acids, Phosphates of potassium and Mg, Nicotinic acid or Riboflavin. It should ideally have the following criteria—

- It should be able to support the growth of moderately exacting bacteria, only from small inoculum.
- It should have a low content of contaminating bacteria.
- It should have a very low content of copper.
- It should not have fermentable carbohydrates.
- It should be Hygroscopic in nature.

CASEIN HYDROLYSATE:

It is a type of amino acid which is obtained by hydrolysis of the milk protein, Casein. It is rich in Phosphates, salts and Growth factors. It also contains Proteolytic enzymes like Trypsin. Tryptophan is destroyed during hydrolysis, under the action of Trypsin and some amino acids are also reduced. It is mainly used as a nearly defined medium, for experimental purpose.

BLOOD *as constituent of the culture media*:

Careful aseptic precautions are to be followed while using blood as a constituent of the culture media. Bacterial contamination should also be excluded. The blood has to be screened for any infections like HIV; HBSAg; HEP C, etc. Blood with glucose is unsuitable. The blood which is non-coagulated only, should be used. The blood can be made not to get coagulated either by defibrination or by adding citrate or oxalate. Defibrination can be done in a sterile bottle with glass beads. The sterile bottle has to be stoppered and used. If it is shaken continuously for 5 minutes, defibrination occurs. There are two types in which blood can be used in the culture media—

   a. *Oxalated blood*: It is prepared by mixing 10ml of 10% solution of neutral potassium oxalate per liter of blood.

   b. *Citrated blood*: It is prepared by mixing 60mg of sodium citrate per 10ml of blood.

The various sources from which blood to be used as / in the culture media, can be obtained, are—

   —Sterile horse blood
   —Rabbit blood
   —Oxen blood
   —Sheep blood

—Human blood

USE: It is used for testing a bacterium which is sensitive to a wide range of antibiotics (Antibiotic Susceptibility Testing).

SERUM: Apart from the above, serum can also be used as an important ingredient in the culture media, as it is a good source of nutrition. It can be either commercially available, or it can be made from defibrinated or oxalated blood. It is sterilized and filtered by Seitz's filter, and can be stored at 3-5°C.

MEAT EXTARCT: It is also an important ingredient in the culture media. It can be commercially prepared by hot water extraction of lean meat, concentrated by evaporation. (Ex: Lab Lemco, Oxioid Unipath).

Apart from the above other sources of nutrition which are also important in the culture media are—

- Yeast extract
- Malt extract p*H ADJUSTMENT*: The pH adjustment can be checked and adjusted by using—pH meters pH indicator dyes
- Lovibonds comparator

EQUIPMENT: The equipment which are mainly required in the preparation of the culture media are—

a. Conical Flasks: They are used to store and melt the

various ingredients of the culture medium which has to be prepared. (Figure 1)

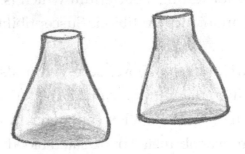

Figure 1 Conical flasks

b. Petri dishes: They are also called as Petri plates. They are used to pour the prepared media (Figure 2). But the media in the petri dishes can deteriorate within one week. So, they are to be immediately used. The petri dish provides a large surface for isolation and observation of colonies. The sample is streaked on the media in the petri plate by using a sterile loop or a sterile swab (Figure 3). It is important that the sterilized loop be cooled before picking up the sample.

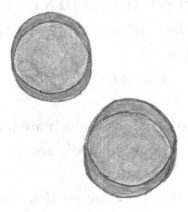

Figure 2 Petri dishses

c. *Test Tubes*: Apart from the above, the test tubes are also used to prepare and store the Culture media (Figure 4). They are also used for transportation of the media. The test tubes are also used for preparing the slants of the culture media for culturing certain organisms like yeasts. They can also be used for storing the cultures, for any further usage. e.g., *Loeffler's Serum Slope.*

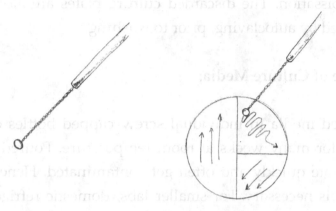

Figure 3 Sterile loop, and sample streaking
on Petri plate using loop

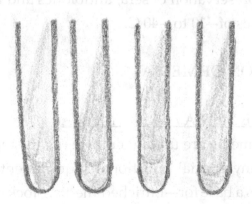

Figure 4 Test tubes with slants

Sterilization of Culture Media:

The Culture media are sterilized in an autoclave at 121°C for 15' under 15 lbs of Pressure. Heat-labile substances like serum and sugar solutions must be sterilized by free-steam or filtration. Egg containing media, like Lowenstein-Jensen's medium, and Loeffler's serum slope medium are sterilized by inspissation. The discarded culture plates are also to be sterilized by autoclaving, prior to washing.

Storage of Culture Media:

Prepared media in individual screw capped bottles can be stored for many weeks at room temperature. Poured plates deteriorate quickly and often get contaminated. Hence, cold storage is necessary. For smaller labs, domestic refrigerators can be used. But for larger labs, insulated cold room with temperatures at 4-5°C has to be used. Deep freeze refrigerators are used for preservation of sera, antibiotics and amino acids, at temperatures of—10 to—40°C.

PREPARATION OF MEDIA:

A. SIMPLE MEDIA / BASAL MEDIA:
   These media are used to culture organisms that do not have any special nutritional requirements. These are used as a base for—Enriched media, Stock cultures, and also for biochemical and serological identification. e.g:

1. Peptone water
2. Nutrient broth
3. Nutrient agar

1. Peptone water is prepared by adding 10 gms of 1% peptone in 5 gms of 0.5% Nacl.

2. Nutrient broth is prepared by adding 1-2% of meat extract to the above said mixture of Peptone water. The meat extract is obtained by meat infusion using lean meat, to which Peptone water is added. The Digest broth is prepared from extract of lean meat which is digested by proteolytic enzymes. It is sterilized by autoclaving at 121ºC for 15 min. Its pH is maintained at 7.2-7.6. it has to be stored in a cool, dark place.

3. Nutrient agar is prepared by adding 2%agar to the above mixture of Nutrient broth. Blood agar is obtained by adding 5% blood to this mixture.

COMPLEX MEDIA:

1. **ENRICHED MEDIA:** These media are used to meet the exact growth requirements of some fastidious bacteria by adding—Blood, Serum, Egg, Yeast extract, Vitamins and Growth factors. They are used to identify and grow organisms from specimens of a normally sterile site. e.g.—Blood agar, Blood broth; Serum agar, Serum broth; Serum peptone water; Chocolate agar; Lysed blood agar; Fildes agar and broth; Glucose agar and broth; Todd Hewitt meat infusion broth; Mueller-Hinton agar.

BLOOD AGAR: It is prepared by melting sterile blood (5-10%), and sterile nutrient agar which are then cooled at 50°C. during melting we should avoid formation of bubbles. It is then stored at 2-8°C, preferably in plastic bags. Blood agar has a shelf life of up to 4 weeks. Layered blood agar is prepared by adding 8ml of Nutrient agar, followed by 8ml of Blood. Thinner blood layer enables hemolytic reaction to be seen more clearly. This medium has a pH range of 7.2-7.6.

USES:

- To differentiate Staphylococcus aures from Staphylococcus epidermidis.
- To identify Vibriocholera, Streptococci.
- Also used for Sensitivity testing.

CHOCOLATE AGAR: It is nothing but heated blood agar. The RBC which are lysed on heating the blood, liberate the nutrients. It is prepared by heating the blood agar at 70°C in a water bath, for about 10-15 min. RBC are lysed at this temperature. Then, at 45°C, it is remixed and dispensed.

LYSED AGAR: It consists of 100 ml of Nutrient agar and about 10-20ml of lysed blood. It is prepared by first melting the nutrient agar, and then, cooling it to 50°C. To this, the lysed blood is added. Then, it is again heated to 55-56°C for approximately 1hour. Then, it is freezed and thawed alternatively. Then, it is treated with saponin.

Use: This medium is used for the growth of Haemophilus infulenzae; Nisseria meningititidis; Streptococcus pneumoniae; and also for the Subculture of Gonococci.

SERUM AGAR and SERUM BROTH: Serum agar is prepared by adding 10%sterile serum with sterile nutrient agar, which is melted and cooled at 55ºC. Likewise, the Serum broth is obtained by boiling 10%sterile serum (sterilized by Seitz filter) with sterile nutrient broth, and then cooling it.

FILDES AGAR and BROTH: Fildes peptic digest of blood is added to nutrient broth or agar, in the proportion of 2-5%, after heating at 55ºC for 30 min, to remove chloroform. Its use stimulates the growth of Hemophillus species.

2. SELECTIVE MEDIA:

The selective media are mainly used to isolate the pathogens like Salmonella typhii, which is usually over grown by commensal bacteria like Escherichia coli. They inhibit the growth of other organisms and allow the growth of the wanted pathogens. Substances with stimulatory effect or inhibitory effect are incorporated in the medium. Some such substances are—Bile salts, chemicals, dyes, antibiotics. The selective media are mainly used for isolating those specimens from a site which usually has normal microbial flora.

Examples of Selective media are—Neomycin Blood Agar; Gentamycin Blood Agar; Wilson and Blair medium, which is highly selective for *Salmonellae*; Lowenstein Jensen medium for *Mycobacterium tuberculosis*; Leifson's deoxycholate—citrate agar (DCA) is a selective differential medium for *Samonellae* and *Shigellae*; Thiosulphate citrate bile sucrose agar is selective for *Vibrio cholerae*.

THIOSULPHATE CITRATE BILE SUCROSE AGAR: It is a highly selective medium. It is prepared by adding Yeast extract + peptone water +sodium citrate+ sodium thiosulphate + NaCl + ox bile + sucrose +bromo thymol blue+ agar. It has a pH of 8.6. It is used for—Isolation of Vibrios; to differentiate sucrose fermenters which develop as yellow colonies, from non-sucrose fermenters, which grow as green colonies. Eg:To differentiate V.cholerae from V.parahemolyticus.

3. ENRICHMENT MEDIA:

These are the liquid media which are used to enhance the growth of a particular organism and suppress the growth of others. e.g.:—Alkaline peptone water

- —Hartley's broth
- —Liver infusion broth
- —Bile broth
- —Tetrathionate broth
- —Selenite F broth

SELENITE F BROTH: Sodium selenite inhibits Coliform bacilli, while permitting the growth of Salmonella and many Shigella spp. It is prepared by adding 5gm peptone + 4gm lactose + 4gm Sodium hydrogen selenite + 9.5gm Disodium hydrogen phosphate + 0.5gm Sodium dihydrogen phosphate, with 1 liter of sterile water. The medium can be sterilized by steam for 20 min at 100 °C, but it should not be autoclaved. It has a pH of 7.1. Since selenite salts are toxic and teratogenic, careful precautions must be observed while handling them.

TETRATIONATE BROTH:

1. The important solutions of this medium—Thiosulphate and Iodine solutions are prepared separately and added later to the medium. Mix 24.8gm of Sodium thiosulhphate salt and 100ml of sterile water, and steam for 30 min at 100°C. This gives the Thio sulphate solution. The Iodine solution contains 20gm of Potassium iodide + 12.7gm of Iodine, and sterile water. First, dissolve the potassium iodide in 50 ml of water. Then, add the iodine and make up to 100ml i.e., 0.5mol per liter solution.

2. The other ingredients which are to be added to the above solutions are—2.5gm Calcium carbonate + 78ml Nutrient broth + 4ml of Iodine sol + 15ml of Thiosulphate sol + 3ml of Phenol red (0.002% in 20%ethanol).

3. The Calcium carbonate is first added to the broth. Then, it is autoclaved for 20min at 121°C. Then, gradually cool it and add Thiosulphate and Iodine solutions, Phenol red solution and mix thoroughly. Then, dispense the medium in screw capped bottles.

   USE:—Enriches Salmonella typhi, Shegellae and inhibits Coliforms.

4. **DIFFERENTIAL MEDIA:** These are the media that show a visible change, as a result of metabolic activity.

e.g.—Mac conkey agar for Lactose fermentors and Non-Lactose fermentors.

MAC CONKEY AGAR: It is used for the cultivation of *Enterobacteriaceae*. It consists of 20gm of Peptone + 5gm of Sodium taurocholate + 1 liter of water + 20gm of agar + 3.5ml of Neutral red sol (2%in 50%ethanol) + Lactose (10% aqueous sol) and made up to 100ml (pH 7.5). It is prepared by adding peptone with sodium taurocholate in water by heating. Then, add the agar and dissolve in an autoclave. To this, the agar is added and dissolved in an autoclave. To this, add lactose and neutral red. Then, heat the mixture in free steam (100°C), for 1 hour, then at 115°C for 15 minutes. Then, pour the plates. This gives a distinct reddish brown colour to the medium. Bile salts are added to inhibit non-intestinal bacteria. Lactose, in combination with Neutral red, distinguishes the coliform (LF) Salmonella from Shigella groups (NLF).

5. **INDICATOR MEDIA:** These media help to reveal a particular property of an organism. e.g.:

a. Wilson and Blair medium: In this medium, Sulphite is reduced to sulphide, and because of this property, the colonies of *Salmonella typhi* will show a metallic sheen.

b. Potassium Telurite medium: This medium is used for identifying the *Corynaebacterium diptheriae*, wherein the Potassium telurite is reduced to metallic telurite by diptheriae, thus, producing black colonies.

c. Blood agar: This medium is used for heamolysis reactions which are specific to *Streptococci* species.

d. <u>Nagler's medium</u>: This medium is used for the Lecitinase activity.

5. **TRANSPORT MEDIUM:** These media are devised to maintain the viability of the pathogen and to avoid overgrowth by contaminats. e.g: a. *Stuart's medium* is used for transportation of *Gonococci.* b. *Amies transport medium,* used or transporting *Neisseira gonorrhea.* c. *Pike's medium,* used for transportation of *Streptococcus pyogens, Haemophilus influenza.* d. *Glycerol saline transport medium,* for transporting *Typhoid bacillus.* e. *Cary blair medium,* for transporting *Salmonella, Shigella, Campylobacter* or *Vibrio cholera spp.* f. Deep semi-solid *Thioglycollate medium, Robertson's Cooked Meat medium* (RCM) are also used for transporting mainly the Anaerobic organisms.

STUART'S TRANSPORT MEDIUM: It mainly consists of 1gm of Sodium thioglycollate; 10gm of Sodium glycerophosohate; 0.1gm of Calcium chloride; 4ml of Agar; 4ml of Methylene blue; and 1 liter of distilled water. Stuart's medium contains reducing agents to prevent oxidation. Charcoal is added, to neutralize certain bacterial inhibitors to Gonococci. It is prepared by dissolving all the solids in distilled water at 100°c and adjusting the pH to 7.3-7.4. Then, add methylene blue solution and distribute in bijou bottles, filling nearly full.

Preparation of swabs used in this medium: Take the swabs of absorbent cotton wool on applicator sticks and boil for 5 min in phosphate buffer 0.007mol per lit at a pH of 7.4. Shake off the excess moisture and immerse it in 1% suspension of finely powered charcoal, twirling until the cotton wool is black. Place the swab in oven. Dry and sterilize at 160°C for 90min.

Use—For Gonoccci; H.influenza

AMIE'S TRANSPORT MEDIUM: It is a slight modification of the Stuart's medium. It does not have Sodium glycerophosphate. It consists of 1gm of Sodium thioglycollate (mercaptoacetate); 3gm of Sodium chloride; 0.2gm of Potassium chloride; 0.1gm of Calcium chloride; 0.1gm of Magnesium chloride; 1.15gm of Disodium hydrogen phosphate; 0.2gm of Potassium dihydrogen phosphate; 10gm of finely powdered charcoal; and 4gm of Agar, in 1liter of Distilled water.

Preparation: Dissolve the chemical salts and the agar in the distilled water at 100°c and add charcoal. Check the pH to be at 7.2, and dispense in bijou bottles filled nearly full. Then, autoclave at 121°C for 15 min and allow it to cool. Frequent inversion of the bottles is required during cooling for even distribution of charcoal.

6. **STORAGE MEDIA:** These media are mainly used for storage and maintenance.

   Examples of such media are—Cooked meat broth; Nutrient agar slopes; Semi-solid nutrient agar stabs; Blood agar; Heated blood agar slopes in small screw capped bottles; Egg medium; and Modified Dorset's egg medium, which is good for preserving gram negative bacilli.

7. **ANAEROBIC CULTURE MEDIA:** The best examples of anaerobic culture media are—
   - Robertson's cooked meat medium / broth
   - Thioglycollate broth
   - Anaerobic blood agar

a. **ROBERTSON'S COOKED MEAT MEDIUM:** The contents of this medium are—500gm of Fresh bullock heart; 500ml of water; 1.5ml of Sodium hydroxide. First, mince the fresh bullock heart and place it in alkaline boiling water. Then, Simmer it for 20 minutes. Then, cloth-dry partially and fill it in the bottles. To this, add 500ml of Filtered Infusion Liquid; 2.5gm of Peptone; and finally 1.25gm of Sodium chloride. Later, steam it at 100°C for 20 minutes, add 1ml of pure hydrochloric acid and filter. Bring the pH to 8.2 and again steam it at 100°C for 30minutes. Then, adjust the pH to 7.8. Care should be taken such that the meat depth is at 2.5cm, in about 15 ml of nutrient broth, which has to extend at least 1cm above the meat. For sterilization, it is autoclaved at 121 °C for 20 min. its pH is 7.5.

   <u>Uses</u>: For growing Anaerobes; for preparation of Stock cultures of aerobic organisms; and can also be used as a Recovery medium for spores.

b. **THIOGLYCOLLATE BROTH:** It mainly contains Semisolid agar; A reducing agent; Methylene blue or Resazurin, which acts as an indicator of the oxidation—reduction potential. It also contains the following—5gm of Yeast extract, which is water soluble; 15gm of Casein hydrolysate; 5.5gm of Glucose; 0.5gm of L-cystine; 0.75gm of Agar; 2.5gm of Sodium chloride; 0.5gm of Sodium thioglycolltae (mercaptoacetate); 1ml of Resazurin sodium sol. (1 in 1000), in 1liter of water.

All the ingredients are mixed and dissolved by steaming at 100°C. then, add Thioglycollate and adjust the pH to 7.3. after this, add the resazurin solution and mix thoroughly. Then, cool it at once to 25°C and store in a dark place (25-35°C). Do not use the medium if it has evaporated enough to effect its fluidity.

c. **ANAEROBIC BLOOD CULTURE MEDIUM:** There is a range of media which can be used for blood culture of Anaerobic organisms. The media used are—Brain heart infusion broth; Brain heart infusion broth with cooked meat particles; Thioglycollate broth; Casteneda medium; Saponin broth; Liquid broth.

8. **SUGAR FERMENTATION MEDIA:** The ingredients of this media are—15gm Peptone; 10ml of 0.5%aq acid fuchsin in 1 ml NaOH, which is called—Andrade's indictor; 20gm of the sugar to be tested, in 1liter of water. The medium is prepared by dissolving the peptone and the indicator in 1 liter of water. Later, add 20gm of sugar (glucose, sucrose, lactose and maltose). Distribute 3ml amounts in standard test tubes, and immerse the inverted Durham's tube in it.

6

MICROBIAL NUTRITION

Cells are mainly made up of macromolecules and water. Cells need nutrients and the organisms differ in the types of nutrients they need. Not all nutrients required in the same amounts. Those that are required in large amounts are called *Macronutrients*. Similarly, those that are required in smaller amounts are called *Micronutrients*.

MACRONUTRIENTS:

1. **Carbon:** Most bacteria use organic compounds as a source of carbon. Many of them use carbon-containing compounds like amino acids, fatty acids, organic acids, sugars, nitrogen bases, aromatic compounds, etc., as building blocks, to synthesize the cell components. On a dry weight basis a typical cell is made of about 50% carbon.

   - Different bacteria utilize different compounds, to obtain this Carbon as the source of energy.

a. *Chemoheterotrophic* organisms obtain energy from glucose by glycolysis, fermentation and the *Krebs cycle*.

b. *Chemoheterotrophic* bacteria synthesize some cell components from intermediates in the above pathways.

2. **Nitrogen:** All organisms need Nitrogen to synthesize enzymes, other proteins and nucleic acids. Some organisms obtain Nitrogen from inorganic sources; a few obtain energy from metabolizing inorganic N-containing substances. Many micro-organisms reduce nitrate (NO_3) to amino groups (NH_2) and use the amino groups to make amino acids.

- Many micro-organisms can utilize ammonia as the sole Nitrogen source. Nitrogen fixing bacteria can take up nitrogen directly from the atmosphere. Some can synthesize all 20 amino acids from amino groups. But for some organisms, some amino acids must have to be provided in their growth medium.

- Some fastidious organisms require all 20 amino acids and other building blocks in their growth medium. Many disease causing organisms obtain amino acids from the cells of the humans or other organisms they invade. A typical bacterial cell is 12% nitrogen by weight.

Other macro nutrients are—

3. **Phosphorus:** It is required for the synthesis of nucleic

acids and phospholipids. It can be either inorganic or organic.

4. **Sulphur**: It is usually obtained from inorganic sources (Sulphate or Sulphide). It is mainly required for S—containing amino acids, some vitamins, and co-enzyme A. e.g. Microbes involved in many chemical transformations of sulphur in the environment.

5. **Potassium**: It is required for the enzymes, especially those involved in the protein synthesis.

6. **Magnesium**: It stabilizes ribosomes, cell membranes and nucleic acids. It is also required for the activity of many enzymes.

7. **Calcium**: It is not essential for the growth of many organisms but helps to stabilize the bacterial cell wall. It also plays a key role in the heat stability of endospores.

8. **Sodium**: It is not required by all organisms. Its need often reflects the natural habitat of the organism. e.g. Marine organisms require sodium, and fresh water organisms do not.

9. **Iron**: It plays a key role in cellular respiration. It forms a key component in cytochromes and iron-sulphur proteins which are involved in electron transport. Under anoxic (anaerobic) conditions iron is in $Fe2+$ state, and is soluble. But under aerobic conditions, it is often $Fe3+$ and forms various insoluble minerals. Bacteria have developed iron-binding proteins (siderophores) that solubilise such iron and transport it into the cell. e.g. Hydroxamic acid derivatives. They Chelate $Fe3+$ very strongly. This complex is carried into cell. Because of

this, the iron is split off and hydroxamate exits the cell and repeats the process.

Examples of Siderophores: Enterobactins like Escherichia coli and Salmonella Typhimurium.

MICRO NUTRIENTS (Trace Elements):

- The Micro nutrients are critical to cell function, even if only required in small amounts. Micronutrients are metals. They play a structural role in many enzymes.

Examples include:

Cobalt, Manganese,
Molybdenum, Nickel,
Selenium and Zinc.

GROWTH FACTORS:

Growth Factors are usually available in the form of organic compounds. They are required in very small amounts and only by some cells. They include vitamins, amino acids, purines, pyrimidines. Most micro-organisms can synthesise all of these compounds. But some of them require one or more to be pre-formed in culture environment. Vitamins are the most commonly needed growth factors; most function as parts of co-enzymes. Most commonly required vitamins are Thiamine (Vitamin B_1), Biotin, Pyridoxine (Vitamin B_6) and Cynocobalamine (Vitamin B_{12}).

MICROBIAL GROWTH and THEIR REQUIREMENTS:

Growth, in microbes, is an increase in the number of cells and not an increase in size. Generation usually occurs due to growth by binary fission; (1)Budding; (2) Conidiospores (Actinomycetes); (3) Fragmentation of filaments. Generation time is the time it takes for a cell to divide and the population to be doubled. Most of the microorganisms require about 1-3 hours (E.coli: every 20 min.). By Binary fission, about 100 cells growing for 5 hours, will produce 1,720,320 cells (21 mins. / generation).

BACTERIAL GROWTH CURVE

- When bacteria is seeded into a suitable liquid medium and incubated, its growth follows a definite course. (Table 8 and Figure 5a)

Table 8 showing Bacterial growth phase and their growth pattern

PHASE	GROWTH PATTERN
LAG PHASE	Maximum metabolic activity. But no cell division
LOG PHASE	Rapid cell division. Cells formed is greater. Bacteria stain uniformly. BACTERICIDIAL DRUGS ACTS THIS STAGE

STATIONARY PHASE	Cell division stops due to depletion of nutrients and accumulation of toxic products. STAGE OF BACTEROSTATIC DRUGS.
Decline phase / death phase	Number of viable declines due to cell death. Due to nutritional exhaustion and toxic accumulation, cell death also due to autolytic enzymes.

CHEMICAL REQUIREMENTS:

OXYGEN REQUIREMENTS: Oxygen is essential for obligate aerobes (final electron acceptor in ETC). Oxygen is deadly for obligate anaerobes. This is because—

- Neither gaseous O2, nor the Oxygen which is covalently bound in compounds is poisonous, because they are non-reactive.
- The forms of oxygen that are toxic, are highly reactive oxidizing agents.
- They do damage to cells by oxidizing compounds such as proteins and lipids.

There are four toxic forms of oxygen:

1. *Singlet oxygen* (^{1}O2): This is molecular oxygen with electrons boosted to higher energy state.
2. *Superoxide radicals* (O2$^-$): Some of them form during

incomplete reduction of oxygen in aerobic and anaerobic respiration. They are so reactive that aerobes produce superoxide dismutases, to detoxify them. Anaerobes lack superoxide dismutase and die as a result of oxidizing reactions of superoxide radicals formed in the presence of oxygen.

3. *Peroxide anion* (O_2^{2-}): They are found in hydrogen peroxide H_2O_2. They are formed during reactions which are catalyzed by superoxide dismutase and other reactions. Aerobes contain either catalase or peroxidase, to detoxify peroxide anion. Obligate anaerobes either lack both enzymes or have only a small amount of each.

4. *Hydroxyl radical* (OH^*): It results from ionizing radiation and from incomplete reduction of hydrogen peroxide. It is the most reactive of the four toxic forms of oxygen. It is not a threat to aerobes due to action of catalase and peroxidase. Aerobes also use antioxidants such as vitamins C and E to protect against toxic oxygen products.

Classification of Organisms Based on Oxygen Requirements:

Aerobes: They undergo aerobic respiration.

Anaerobes: They do not use aerobic metabolism.

Facultative anaerobes: They can maintain life via fermentation or anaerobic respiration or by aerobic respiration.

Aerotolerant anaerobes: They do not use aerobic metabolism but have some enzymes that detoxify the poisonous forms of Oxygen.

Microaerophiles: They are the aerobes that require oxygen levels from 2-10% and have a limited ability to detoxify hydrogen peroxide and superoxide radicals.

PHYSICAL REQUIREMENTS FOR MICROBIAL GROWTH:

1. Temperature pH
2. Osmolarity
3. Pressure

1. TEMPERATURE:

Based on the Growth Temperatures, the organisms are divided into (Figure 5a and Figure 5b):

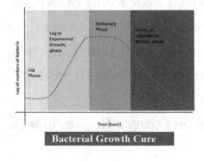

Bacterial Growth Cure

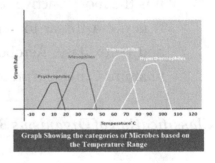

Graph Showing the categories of Microbes based on the Temperature Range

Figure 5a   Figure 5b

Psychrophiles: Optimum temperature for these organisms is 15°C.

Psychrotrophs: Their optimum temperatures range from 20-30°C.

Mesophiles: The optimum temperatures for these organisms range from 25-40°C.

Thermophiles: The optimum temperatures for these organisms range from 50-60°C.

Effect of temperature on proteins—Too high Temperatures cause denaturation of Proteins.

Effect of temperature on lipid-containing membranes of cells and organelles—If the temperatures are too low, membranes become rigid and fragile. If they are too high membranes become too fluid and cannot contain the cellular organelle.

2. pH:

Organisms are sensitive to changes in acidity because H+ and OH-interfere with H bonding in proteins and nucleic acids. Most bacteria grow between pH 6.5 and 7.5 and they are called *Neutrophiles*. Molds and yeasts grow between pH 5 and 6, and are called *Acidophiles*. They grow in acidic environments. *Alkalinophiles* live in alkaline soils and water up to pH 11.5.

3. PHYSICAL EFFECTS OF WATER:

Microbes require water to dissolve enzymes and nutrients, which are required in their metabolism. Water is important reactant in many metabolic reactions. Most cells die in absence of water. Some microbes have cell walls that retain water. Endospores and cysts cease most metabolic activity in a dry environment for years.

There are two physical effects of water—

- Osmotic pressure
- Hydrostatic pressure

- **OSMOTIC PRESSURE:** It is the pressure exerted on a semi-permeable membrane by a solution containing solutes that cannot freely cross membrane. It is more related to concentration of dissolved molecules and ions in a solution.

  - Hypotonic solutions: They have lower solute concentrations. Cells placed in these solutions will swell and burst.

  - Hypertonic solutions: They have greater solute concentrations. Cells placed in these solutions will undergo *Crenation* (shriveling of cytoplasm) / *Plasmolysis*. This effect helps in preserving some foods, and also restricts organisms to certain environments. *Extreme / Obligate halophiles*—grow in up to 30% salt, i.e., they require high osmotic pressure. *Facultative halophiles* can tolerate high salt concentrations (Osmotic pressures).

- *Hydrostatic Pressure*: Water exerts pressure on any surface, in proportion to its depth. For every addition of depth, water pressure increases by 1 atmosphere. Organisms that live under extreme pressure are *Barophiles*. Their membranes and enzymes depend on this pressure to maintain their three-dimensional, functional shape.

7

CENTRIFUGE, COLORIMETER, BACTERIAL COUNT.

"Centrifuge is a Device for separation of microorganism from suspending fluid" (Table 9)

1. Size.   2. Density   3. viscosity.

Table 9 Size, Density and Viscosity characters of Microorganism

1. SIZE An increase in size of particle: Larger particle sediment faster. (i.e., Yeast, fungi > bacteria > Virus)
2. DENSITY An increase in difference between the density of particles: Capsulated bacterium > Non capsulated.

3. VISCOSITY:

Decrease in viscosity sediments faster

Serum samples takes much longer than saline samples

TYPES OF ROTOR—CENTRIFUGE (Table 10)

Table 10: Types of Rotor used in Centrifuge and their principle

TYPE OF CENTRIFUGE	PRINCIPLE	CONDITION
HORIZONTAL SWING ROTOR	Sample bucket freely from vertical to horizontal plane.	Bacterological work.
FIXED ANGLE ROTOR	Sample containers are maintained at fixed angle 20°-45° during rotation	Rate of sedimentation is quicker.
VERTICAL ROTORS	Sample tubes are held in vertical postion. Rotor must be carefully used with acclerator and deceleration	Control of speed is difficult

FACTORS INFLUENCING SEDIMENTATION
WHILE CENTRIFUGE

1. The size of particle.
2. Volume of material.
3. Temperature. (low temperature—this prevents metabolism, loss of vitality or enzyme activity during centrifugation)

Types of tubes and bottles:

Glass, plastic, cellulose nitrate and stainless steel.

Toughened glass tubes and Plastic containers are used for bacterological cultures.

BACTERIAL COUNT (Number and Growth)

A. Number

1. **Total count.**
2. **Viable Count.**

   i. Pour plate method
   ii. Surface viable count by spreading method (Table 11)
   iii. Surface viable count by Miles and misra method. (Table 11)

3. **Photo Electric colorimeter and spectrophotometer.**

1. Total Count

- Fix bacterial suspension by adding 2-3 drops of formalin.
- Wash, rinse, drain and dry the counting chamber and cover slip it.
- Slide counting chamber: Hawksley and gallen kamp: (Figure 6) : thin glass slide with a flat circular platform depressed exactly 0.02mm below the surface / trench. It has engraved lines into 400 small squares (0.0025mm^2)

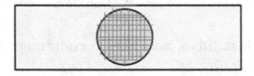

Figure 6 hawksley and gallen kamp

2. Viable count i. Pour plate method

1. Number of living bacteria in liquid culture / suspension is counted by culture method.
2. Suspension (1ml of each dilution) is mixed with molten agar medium (Nutrient agar) in petri dish. Incubate culture for 2 days at 37°C.

Count the colonies in three plates.

Dilution factor

(1 dilution contain 50-500 bacterial / ml).

Table 11: Surface viable count

Surface viable count	
SPREADING METHOD	**MILES and MISRA METHOD.**
Plate of medium is dried, at 37°C for 10-15minutes	Plate of medium is dried, at 37°C for 10-15minutes.
0.02-0.1 ml of dilution is pipetted	Calibrated pipette—each drop, 0.02ml in volume.
Poured over the surface of each three plates and spread widely with sterile glass spreader.	Poured over the surface of 5 plates. Each plate receive one drop.
Viable count = <u>average colony count</u> plate	Colony Counts are made in drop area. Viable count = colony /0.1ml of dilution.

3. <u>**Photo electric colorimeter and spectrophotometer:**</u>

    1. Most accurate method, measures the quantity of micro organism depends on turbidity (opaqueness).

    2. Based on depth of color in solution.

    3. Much quicker, avoid manual error.

    4. Automatic scanning instruments.

3. **Growth (Table 12)**

Table 12: Bacterial growth by wet and dry weight

Wet weight	Dry weight	Total nitrogen
The moist surface growth on a solid medium is scraped and weighed once. Inaccurate— difficulty of evaluating the relative contribution of water wetting the bacterial surface.`	The weight of dried solid matter of bacteria is better to measure of their protoplasm.	Most reliable and constant method for measuring the bacterial protoplasm. "Estimate the nitrogen present in the nitrogenous components of the cells." (N_2 content = 16%)
	The cells from known volume of culture are centrifuged. The weight of centrifuged cells weighed. Weighed again after drying by placing over hot air oven.	The cells from known volume of culture are centrifuged. Cells + H_2so_4+ $CuSo_4$—K_2So_4— selenium catalyst.-→ ammonium nitrate is produced Ammonium nitrate is trapped and measured by nessler's reagent.

Turbidity

Turbidity of a suspension is caused by light scattered by particulate matter during the passage through the suspension.

1. By measuring the amount of light scattered directly— nepelometry (rarely practiced)
2. By measuring the light lost from the beam by scattering.

8

IMMUNOLOGICAL AND SEROLOGICAL METHODS IN MICROBIOLOGY

An antibody is an immunoglobulin molecule secreted into the tissue fluids from lymphoid cells, which have exposed to a foreign substance—an antigen.

1. PRECIPITATION—(Immunodiffusion, Immunoelectrophoresis, counter current electrophoresis.)
2. AGGLUTINATION—(Haemagglutination, Tube and Slide agglutination, Passive agglutination.)
3. COMPLEMENT FIXATION

1. PRECIPITATION

i. IMMUNODIFFUSION

1. Antibody is incorporated in to agar gel.
2. Different dilutions of antigen are placed in holes punched in to the agar. (Figure 7)

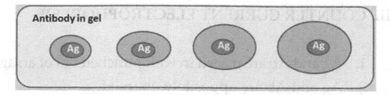

Figure 7 Immunodiffusion

3. Antigen diffuses in to gel, it reacts with antibody and when the equivalence point is reached, ring of precipitation is formed.
4. Ring is proportional to the log of the concentration of antigen.

ii. IMMUNOELECTROPHORESIS

1. A complex mixture of antigens is placed in a well punched out of an agar gel.
2. Antigens are electrophoresed—so that antigen are separated according to their charge.
3. After electrophoresis, a trough is cut in the gel and antibodies are added.
4. As antibodies diffuse in to agar, a precipitin lines are produced in the zone. (Figure 8)

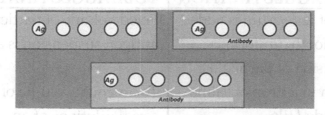

Figure 8 Immunoelectrophoresis

iii. COUNTER CURRENT ELECTROPHORESIS

1. Ag and Ab are placed in well punched out of an agar.
2. Ag and Ab are oppositely charged.
3. Subjected to electrophoresis, they form of precipitation line, even thickness of precipitation line also quantitative. (Figure 9)

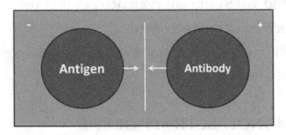

Figure 9 Counter current electrophoresis

2. AGGLUTINATION

—Slide and Tube agglutination methods are represented in table 13.

Table 13: Slide and Tube agglutination.

SLIDE AGGLUTINATION	TUBE AGGLUTINATION
Drop of antiserum is added to a smooth, uniform suspension of particulate antigen in a drop of saline on a slide / tile.	Fixed volume of particulate antigen suspension is added + To an equal volume of serial dilutions of an antiserum in test tubes

| | Eg: Widal test. |
| | Paul Bunnel test. |

III.PASSIVE AGGLUTINATION

1. The only difference between the requirements for precipitation and agglutination test is the physical nature of antigen.
2. By attaching soluble Ag's to surface of carrier particle, it is possible to convert the ppt test into agglutination test
3. More convienent and more sensitive in detection of antibodies.
4. Called as passive agglutination (Figure 10).

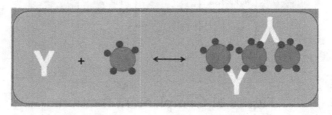

Figure 10 Passive agglutination

Commonly used carrier particle—red cell (Human / sheep) or latex particle / bentonite.

Eg:
1. Rose waaler test—RA.
2. TPHA—syphillis
3. Detection of antibodies to viral antigens.

3. COMPLEMENT FIXATION

Complement takes part in many immunological reactions and is absorbed during the combination of antigens with their antibodies.

In presence of appropriate antibodies, complement lyses erythrocytes.

Eg: WASSERMAN 'S TEST

Complement Fixation : (Figure 11)

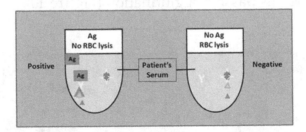

Figure 11 Complement fixation

Step: 1

1. Inactivation of patient's serum by heating at 56˚c for half hour. This causes destruction of the complement activity in serum.
2. Addition of Soluble / particulate antigen.
3. Addition of guinea pig "complement"
   If serum contains antibody, complement will be utilized for antigen—antibody interaction.
   If serum contains no antibody, No Antigen—Antibody interaction will happen. Complement will be left intact.

Step: 2

4. Add sensitized sheep red cell (MHD)

   Negative: Lysis of red cell indicate—complement was not used in first step.

   Positive: Absence of red cell lysis; complement was used in first step.

9

IDENTIFICATION, MORPHOLOGY, STAINING, SPECIES VARIATION AND LABORATORY DIAGNOSIS OF BACTERIA:

S.No.	TOPIC
1.	Introduction
2.	To Differentiate The Gram Positive Cocci Organisms. 1. CATALASE TEST
3.	Differentiation of Catalase and Gm positive, Staphylococci and Micrococci. 1. Modified Oxidase test 2. Oxidation—Fermentation Test 3. Furasolidine and Bacitracin Susceptibility Test.

4.	Staphylococcus
	1. Morphology, Toxin, Enzymes by it and varies species of staphylococcus.
	2. Culturing technique, Colony Morphology, Microscopic character and Gm staining property.
	3. Species variation identification of staphylococcus b/n S. aureus and epidermidis and Saphrophyticus.
	i. Coagulase Test.
	ii. Mannitol Fermentation Test.
	iii. DNAse Test.
	iv. Hemolysis on Blood Agar.
5.	Streptococcus
	1. Morphology and characterstic of Streptococcus.
	2. Classification.
	3. Classification of S. Viridans based on Biochemical characterstics.
	4. Lancefield classification
	5. Toxins and Enzymes.
	6. Culture Techniques, characterstics, Microscopic appearance and Gm staining property.
	7. Test carried for Alpha—Hemolytic Streptococci.
	1. Optochin susceptibility Test.

	A. Differentiation of S. Viridans, Pneumoniae, Enterococcus.
	1. Bile solubility Test
	2. Bile Aesculin Test.
	8. Test Carried for Beta—Hemolytic Streptococci.
	1. Bacitracin—SXT Test
	2. PYR Test
	3. CAMP Test
6.	Actinomyces.
	1. Morphology, culture Technique and characterstics, Gm Staining property.
	2. Laboratory test for Actinomyces Isralei
7.	Mycobacterium
	1. Morphology, classification.
	2. Identification of M. Tuberculosis.
	3. Aryl Sulphatase Test.
	4. Tuberculin, Mantoux and Heaf Test.
	Treponema
	1. Morphology, characterstics of T. palladium.
	2. Laboratory diagnosis of Syphillis.
	3. Choice of serological Test for syphilis.
	Sensitivity and Specificity of Various Serological test for Syphilis.

IDENTIFICATION, MORPHOLOGY, STAINING, SPECIES VARIATION AND LABORATORY DIAGNOSIS OF BACTERIA

INTRODUCTION

Bacteria are classified in to Gram positive and negative based on Gram's staining. This acts as primary technique to employ in the identifying the morphology of bacteria. Later based on its shape it is classified in to cocci and bacilli, spirella, spirocheate.

TO DIFFERENTIATE THE GRAM POSITIVE COCCI ORGANISMS:

CATALASE TEST: (Figure 12)

Take few test colonies with glass/ plastic (avoid iron loop)

Drop the stick in test tube containing 0.5-1ml H_2O_2

The results are observed based on bubble formation (Table 13)

The control usage in the catalase test are shown in table 14.

Table 13 showing the results of catalase test based on the bubble formation

Immediate bubble formation	Positive
No bubble formation	negative

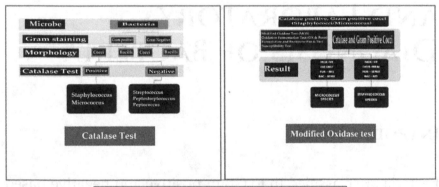

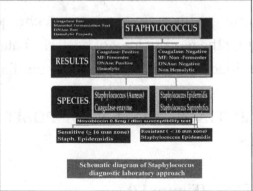

Figure 12 Catalase text, Modified Oxidase test and schematic diagram of staphylococcus diagnostic laboratory approach.

Table 14: controls in the catalase test

Positive	Staphylococcus
Negative	streptococcus

MODIFIED OXIDASE TEST (Figure 12)

Differentiates micrococcus species from other gram positive coccus.

1. Filter paper is soaked with 6% tetramethyl p phenylene diamine dihydrochloride in dimethyl sulfoxide (DMSO)
2. Place the filter paper on slide.
3. Take the test colony and smear it on the filter paper.
4. Results: (Table 15)

Table 15: Results for Modified Oxidase test

Appearance of dark blue colonies in 2 minutes	Positve
NO change in colour in 2 minutes	Negative

Table 16: Control in Modified oxidase test

Micrococcus species	Positive control
Staphylococcus aures species	Negative control

Furazolidine—Bacitracin test

This test helps to differentiate the micrococci with streptococci (Table 17)

1. Inoculate the organism from culture to sheep blood supplemented—mueller hinton agar (beef infusion,+ Casein hydrolysate+ starch+ Agar+ distill water) plate in 3 directions.
2. Place 0.04 μg Bacitracin and 100 μg Furazolidone disc on surface of plate.

Table 17: showing results to furazolidine and bacitracin disc usage.

Genus	Furazolidine	Bacitracin
Micrococcus	Resistant	Sensitive
Staphylococcu	Sensitive	resistant

OXIDATIVE—FERMENTATIVE TEST (Figure 12)

- This test Differentiates Organisms that oxidises the carbohydrates (micrococcus) to organisms that ferments the carbohydrates. (staphylococcus)
1. Test colonies are inoculated to bottom of two tubes of Hugh and lefson media(dipottasium hydrogen phosphate+Nacl+peptone+agar+bromothymol+water)
2. Cover the inoculum with liquide paraffin 1cm deep in one of the tube.

3. Incubate up to 14 days at 37°c up to 14 days.
4. Results are shown in table 18

Table 18: showing the results of oxidase fermentation test:

Open tube	Closed/ sealed tube	Interpretation
Yellow	Green	Oxidative organism
Yellow	Yellow	Fermentative org.

STAPHYLOCOCCUS

1. Gm positive, catalase positive, MOX negative, oxidative and fermentative, non—motile, non—sporing, clustering cocci.
2. Cluster formation is due to sequential division of bacteria in three perpendicular planes.
3. Staph auerus posses capsule and inhibit phagocytosis. Capsule : peptidoglycan and teichoic acid is antigenic determinant of staph.
4. Toxins of staphylococcus are shown in table 19.
5. Enzymes of staphylococcus organism are shown in table 20.
6. Microbiology study details of staphylococcus aureus are shown in table 21.

Table 19: Toxins of Staphylococcus

TOXIN
Alpha : strongly active on Rabbit red cells (most important pathogenicity)
Beta: lysis of sheep red cells
Gamma and delta : acts on human, horse, sheep and rabbit red cell
Leucocidin : (Panton—valentine toxin) : lysis of white cells
Enterotoxin : food posioning.
Toxic shock syndrome toxin (diarrhoea, vomit, high fever, Hyper tension)
Epidermolytic toxin.

Table 20: Enzymes in staphylococcus organism

Enzyme
Coagulase: (heat labile) It has property to clot human or rabbit plasma. CRF(coagulase reactive factor) is present in rabbit and human plasma. Coagulase converts fibrinogen into fibrin. Clumping factor (bound coagulase—heat stable—clumping in cocci, precipitates fibrin on the cell surface)
Different species

S. Aureus (H)	
S. intermedius.	
S. Hyicus	
S. Epidermidis(H)	
S. Capitis(H)	
S. Hominis(H) weak	
S. Warneri	
S. Hemolytics(H) weak	
S. Cohni (H) weal	
S. Saprophytics(H)	

Table 21: Showing the Microbiological details of Staphylococcus Auerus.

PATHOGEN	COLONY MORPHOLOGY (AFTER OVERNIGHT INCUBATION AT 37°c	MICROSCOPIC MORPHOLOGY	STAINING REACTION	SAMPLE
STAPH. AUREUS	BLOOD AGAR: Smooth 1-2 mm diameter cream / white, slightly raised occasionally. hemolytic colonies. (Figure 12) Mannitol salt agar: Yellow colored colonies with yellow zone	Coccus in irregular cluster, Singly or in pair, uniform size and non motile	Gm +ve	Pus, sputum, Blood, fecus, vomit, urine, food.

COAGULASE TEST (Table 22)

Table 22: Slide and tube coagulation test in Staphylococcus

Slide coagulation (bound Coagulase)	Tube coagulation test (free coagulase)
A few colonies of bacteria are add to a drop of saline on clean glass slide. Mix the rabbit or human plasma. Clumping shows positive	0.1ml of an over night broth culture is mixed with 0.5ml of human / rabit plasma. In tube 2: dilute plasma alone control Tube incubated in water bath at 37°C for 3-6 hours Plasma clots in positive.
	Positive—S. aureus Negative—staph epidermidis / saprophyltics.

Mannitol fermentation test (Figure 12)

- Inoculate the organism from the culture to mannitol agar medium (nutrient agar with 1% mannitol + Nacl + Phenol as indicator)
- Test result are analysed by colour changes (table 23.)

Table 23: Results of Mannitonal fermentation test

Yellow colored colonies	Positive (staph. Aureus)
No color change	Negative

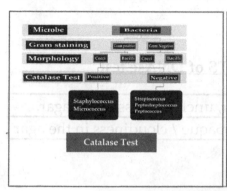

Catalase Test

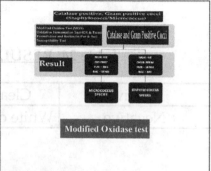

Modified Oxidase test

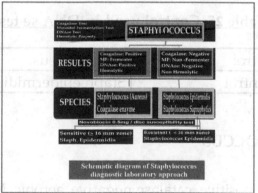

Schematic diagram of Staphylococcus diagnostic laboratory approach

DNAse TEST

- This test helps to differentiate the staphylococcus aureus with other species of staph and micrococcus.

1. Inoculate the organism from culture on DNA agar plate.
2. Incubate the medium at 37°C.
3. Flood the medium with few drops of 3.6 % Hcl.

4. After few minutes examine the plate against dark background.
5. Test results are analyzed by the changes in the agar medium (table 24)
6. Controls used in the DNAse test are shown in table 25

Table 24: RESULTS of DNAse test

Positive	Clear, uncloudiness in the agar.
Negative	White opaque / cloudiness in the agar

Table 25: Control used in DNA se test

Positive control	Staph aureus
Negative control	Staph epidermidis.

STREPTOCOCCUS

1. Gram positive, catalase negative, aerobic, Non—motile, Non—sporing cocci arranged in chains. (Figure 13)
2. Chain formation due to successive cell division in one plane only.
3. Capsule inhibits phagocytosis.
4. Cell wall contains protein s M, T and R which are antigenic determinant sites.
5. Biochemical characterization of streptococcus is shown in Figure 13.

Serological group	Species	Habitat
A	S.Pyogenes	Human
B	S. Agalactiae	Human, cattle
C	S. Dysga;actoae, equi, equisimilis, zoo epidemicus	Human, Cattle, horse, animals
D	S. Fecalis, fecum, durans, avium,bovis, equinus	Man, Birds, feces of horses.
E,P,U,V	S. Infrequens	Pigs, cattle
F,G	S. Anginosus	Man
H	S. Sanguis	Mouth &intestine of Man
K	S. Salivaris(alpha)	Mouth & intestine of Man
L	S. Salivaris (ß)	Dogs & pigs
M	S. Salivaris (alpha or Non – hemolytic)	Dogs
N	S. Lactis, cremoris	Milk & dairy products
O	S. Cremoris	Man
Q	S. Avium	Birds
R,S,T	S.suis	Pigs

Lance Field Classification of Streptococcus

Figure 13 Classification of Streptococcus, and Biochemical characterization of Streptococcus.

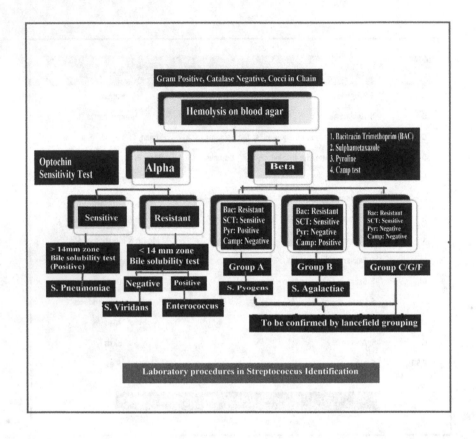

Laboratory procedures in Streptococcus Identification

6. Lance field categorization of streptococcus is shown in figure 14.
7. Laboratory identification of Streptococcus is shown in figure 14.
8. Streptococcal toxins are shown in table 26
9. Microbiological details of Streptococcus pyogens and streptococcus viridians are shown in table 27

Table 26:Streptococcal Toxins

Toxins
1. Hemolysin :   Streptolysin O and S (O : Oxygen labile)   Streptolysis O   It is inactivated in pressence of oxygen.   It is lysis of RBC, cytotoxic for neutrophil, platelets, cardiac tissue.   (> ASO titre in serum is excess of 200 units— streptococcal infection)   Streptolysis S   Oxygen stable   Responsible for hemolysis around the colonies in blood agar plates.   2. Pyrogenic exotoxin: Toxin responsible for rash in scarlet fever.   This toxin injected in to skin of a susceptible child— erythematous reaction—Dick test.   In scarlet fever, antitoxin is injected locally in to rash, blanching of rash seen called schultz charlton reaction.
Enzymes: 1. Streptokinase :   Lysis of human fibrin clot by conversion of plasminogen in to plama—spread of infection.   2. Hyaluronidase: breaks hyaluronic acid of tissue— favours spread of streptococcal lesion.

Table 27: Microbiological details of Streptococcus Pyogens and Viridans

Pathogen	Colony morphology after incubation at 37°C	Microscopic	Gm staining
S. Pyogenes	1. <u>Blood agar :</u> Circular, discrete, semi— transparent, low convex, beta hemolysis. 2. <u>Mc conkey's agar :</u> No colony appear. 3. <u>Enriched broth :</u> Granular deposit, supernatant clear.	Non capsulated occurs in long chains from smear in fluid culture but preparatipm	Gm+ve.
S. Viridans	Blood agar : Small convex colonies and have zone of partial hemolysis and greenish—alpha	Non capsulated, Non—motile Cocci in short chains	Gm +ve

OPTOCHIN SUSCEPTIBILITY TEST

1. This test differentiates Streptococcus pneumonia with other species.
2. Streak one quardant of 5% sheep blood agar with inoculum.
3. Place optochin disc (ethyl hydrocuprein) in centre of inoculum.
4. Incubate 35°c-37°c over night.
5. Results of Optochin susceptibility test interpretation is shown in table 28.

Table 28: Interpretation of Optochin susceptibility test results:

Zone > 14 mm	Sensitive
Zone < 14mm	Resistant.

BILE SOLUBILITY TEST

1. This test differentiates between bile souluble (S.Pneumoniae) with bile insolublers (S. Viridans)
2. Add test colonies in a tube with saline, gives as turbid suspension.
3. Divide suspension into 2 tubes.
4. Add 2 drops of sodium deoxycholate (100g/l) in one tube
5. Add distill water in another tube.
6. Wait 10-15 mts.
7. Results of bile solubility test interpretation are shown in table 29.

Table 29:Interpretation of Bile solubility test results

Clearing of turbidity	Positive (S.pneumoniae)
No clearing of turbidity	Negative

BILE AESCULIN TEST

- This test differentiates between enterococcus with non enterococcus (S. Viridans)

1. Inoculate the organism in bile aesculin agar
2. Incubate at 44°c-45°c for 1-2 hrs.
3. Results of bile aesculin test interpretation are shown in table 30.

Table 30:Interpretation of Bile Aesculin test results

Color of medium changes to black color	Positive
NO color change	Negative (S. Viridans)

Bacitracin and SXT Sensitivity test

- Identifies the S. Pyogenes (group A streptococcus)

1. Streak the half of 5% sheep blood agar plate with inoculum.
2. Place one bacitracin disc (0.04µ/ disc) ; One SXT (sulphamethoxazole 23.75µg) in centre of inoculum.

3. Incubate at 37°C over night.
4. Results of Bacitracin and SXT Sensitivity test interpretation are shown in table 31.

Table 31:Interpretation of Bacitracin and SXT Sensitivity test results

Growth greater than 15mm in diameter zone	Sensitive
Growth only up to the edge of disc	Resistant.

PYR test (Pyrrolidonyl pepitdase)

- Differentiate St. pyogenes with other St. variants

1. Rub a small amount of colony over the filter paper impregentated with pyrrolidonyl pepitdase ß napthylamide.
2. Add dimethyl aminocinnamaldehyde
3. Observe with in 5 minutes
4. Results of PYR test interpretation are shown in table 32.

Table 32:Interpretation of PYR test results

Bright red color change in 5 minutes	Positive test
No color change	Negative.

CAMP TEST

(christie Atkins Munch Peterson)

- Differentiates Group B Streptococcus With Other Group Streptococcus

1. Over 10% sheep blood agar medium.
2. Streak the known strain of staph aureus.
3. Streak a known Enterococcus Rt angle to S. aureus streak with out touching.
4. Streak the test organism Rt. Angle to S. aureus streak with out touching.
5. Results of CAMP test interpretation are shown in table 33.

Table 33: Interpretation of CAMP test results

Enhanced hemolysis of test organism with an arrow shaped area	Positive (Group B)
No enhanced hemolysis of test organism with an arrow shaped area.	Non Group B streptococcus

LACTOBACILLUS

1. Gram positive, non—motile, non—sporing, anaerobic bacilli, form considerable amount of lactic acid from carbohydrates and grow best at pH5.

Saliva sample

{lactobacillus count for DC}

1. Mix patient saliva with 10cc of sterile saline.
2. Add 0.1ml Over the Nutritive broth with kulp's tomato peptone agar plate.
3. Incubate the plate under anerobic condition at 37°C for 3-4days.
4. Count the colonies.
5. More than 10^5 Lactobacillus / ml of saliva is indicative of caries activity.

CARIES ACTIVITY and SUSCEPTIBILITY TEST

TERMINOLOGIES:

CAREIS ACTIVITY TEST:

Measures the degree to which the local environment changes favours the probability of cariouslesions.

CARIES ACTIVITY:

Increment of active lesions over a stated period of time.

CARIES SUSCEPTIBILITY:

Inherent tendency of the host, the target tissue, i.e., the tooth to be afflicted by the caries.

1. LACTOBACILLUS TEST

- Mix patient saliva with 10cc of sterile saline.
- Add 0.1ml Over the Nutritive broth with kulp's tomato peptone agar plate.
- Incubate the plate under anerobic condition at 37°C for 3-4days.
- Count the colonies.
- More than 10^5 Lactobacillus / ml of saliva is indicative of caries activity.

2. SALIVARY REDUCTASE TEST

- Measures the activity of reductase enzyme.
- Saliva sample is added to solution containing diazoresorcinol. Changes from blue to red to color less. (Table 34)

Table 34: Color changes in Salivary reductase test and their interpretation on caries activity

COLOR	TIME	SCORE	CARIES ACTIVITY
BLUE	15 MIN	1	NON CONDUCIVE
ORCHID	15 MIN	2	SLIGHTLY CONDUCIVE
RED	15 MIN	3	MODERATELY CONDUCIVE

| RED | IMMEDIATELY | 4 | HIGHLY CONDUCIVE |
| PINK / WHITE / COLORLESS | IMMEDIATELY | 5 | EXTREMELY CONDUCIVE |

3. SNYDER TEST:

Stimulated saliva is inoculated into glucose and agar containing media, bromocresol green : pH 4.7-5.0(blue green) to 4 (yellow). (Table 35)

Table 35: Snyder test interpretation

Time in hours	24	48	72
Color	Yellow	Yellow	Yellow
Caries activity	Marked	Definite	Limited
Color	Green	Green	Green
Caries activity	Highly susceptbile	Definitely susceptible	Non— susceptible

ACTINOMYCES

1. Gram positive, non—motile, non sporing, non—AF filamentous organism, they often grow in mycelial forms and break up in to coccal and bacillary forms.

2. Laboratory procedures in Actinomyces identification is shown in figure 15.
3. Microbiological details of Actinomyces is shown in table 36.

Table 36: Microbiological details of Actinomyces

Pathogen	Colony morphology	Microscopic morphology	Gm staining
Actinomyces	Grow under anaerobic condition at 37°c for 5-7 days. Blood agar: Small, cream or grey white nodular surface, entire or lobulated colonies which adhere to medium	Non sporing, Non motile Fragmented thin branching,	Gm +ve

MYCOBACTERIUM

1. Slender, straight or slightly curved with rounded ends, occurs singly or in pairs, non sporing, non motile, non capsulated bacilli often difficult to stain, once stained, resist decolorisation—hence the name Acid Fast Bacilli
2. Laboratory procedures in Mycobacterium tuberculosis identification is shown in figure 15.
3. Culture details of mycobacterium (table 37)
4. Diagnostic test in Tuberculosis (Table 39)

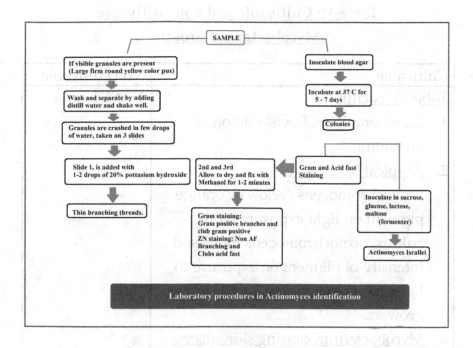

Laboratory procedures in Actinomyces identification

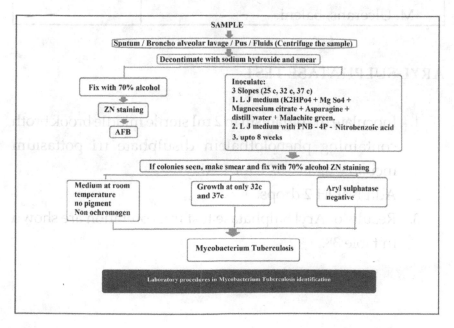

Laboratory procedures in Mycobacterium Tuberculosis identification

Table 37: Cultivable and non cultivable Mycobacterium group.

Cultivable	Non cultivable
Tubercle bacilli: 1. M. tuberculosis, Bovis, microti, africanum. 2. Atypical Mycobacterium: Photochromogens (yelow or orange pigment on light exposure while culture, scotochromogens increased intensity of pigment on exposure to light, Non photochromogens, rapid growers. 3. Mycobacterium causing skin ulcers: M. Ulcerans, baleni.	1. M. Leprae

ARYL SULPHATASE TEST

1. Inoculate the organism in 2 ml sterile middle brook broth containing phenolpthalein disulphate tri pottasium incuabte at 35°c 37°c for 18 days.
2. Add NaOH 2 drops.
3. Results of Aryl Sulphatase test interpretation are shown in table 38.

Table 38: Interpretation of Aryl Sulphatase results

Pink red color	Positive (Rapid growers.)
No color change	Negative (M. tuberculosis)

Table 39: Diagnostic test in Tuberculosis

TUBERCULIN TEST	MANTOUX TEST	HEAF TEST
Demonstrated by Type IV hypersensitivity. Intradermal inj of Tuberculin—(A protein extract from Tubercle bacilli) A positive test—who has not undergone BCG indicates the tuberculous infection recently.	PURIFIED PROTEIN DERIVATIVE (PPD)—{prepared by M. TB grown in semi synthethic media} injected intracutaneously in to akin of fore arm. Examined and palpated after 72 hrs. Firm induration > 10mm is positive If reaction is negative test is reperated with 100 TU.	Done with multiple puncture over skin and a drop of undiluted PPD is spread over the area of skin and pressed Site inspected after 72 hrs. Presence of erythema / oedema / induration atleast in 4 hrs considered as positive.

Not accurate, negative test can also be seen in secondary tuberculosis.	More accurate and used routinely.	Since, needle pack can be used again, contamination of HIV and Hep risk. Not used. Used in epidemological surveys.

TREPONEMA

1. Gram negative, spirochaete, motile, strictly anerobic thin bacteria with tapering ends.
2. Because of it's thinnes, it does't take bacterial stains.
3. It can be negatively stained with india ink.
4. It can't be cultivated.
5. Laboratory diagnostic test in syphilis identification is shown in table 40 a, b and c
6. Choice of available serological test to diagnose syphilis (Table 41)
7. Positive predictive value of diagnostic test in syphilis (Table 42)

Table 40 a: laboratory diagnosis of syphilis

Laboratory diagnosis of syphilis
Demonstration of treponemes
Serological test
Non treponemal test
Treponemeal test

1. **Cardiolipin antigen is an alcoholic extract of beef heart tissue to which lecithin and cholestrol is added— VDRL antigen**

Table 40 b: laboratory diagnosis of syphilis

DFA—TP	Smear of material to be test is made on glass side + Flourescent labelled monoclonal antibody Stained : appears, distinct sharply outlined apple green fluorescence.
VDRL TEST	Slide flocculation test : VDRL ANTIGEN + Reagin—visible clumps : positive
RPR Rapid Plasma Reagin	VDRL antigen suspended in choline chloride mixed with finely divided carbon particles. + patient serum / plasma Clumps : positive

BIOLOGICAL FALSE POSITIVE REACTIONS (BFP):

Cardiolipin is non specific antigen may react with sera of patients who may not have syphillis, accounts for BFP. These includes:

1. Leprosy
2. Malaria
3. Relapsing fever
4. Hepatitis
5. Systemic Lupus Erythematosus.

Table 40 c : laboratory diagnosis of syphilis

TP Immobilisation test (live T. Palladium	Test serum + actively motile Nichol's strain of T. pallidum and incubated anerobically. If antibodies are present the treponema are immobilised when examined under microscope.
Using killed T. palladium 1. TPA	Suspension of T. palladium is inactivated by formalin. This is mixed with test serum and Examined under dark ground microscopy. Treponema agglutinated in presence of antibodies.

2. TPIA	Suspension of inactivated T. palladium is mixed with test serum +complement + Fresh heparinized whole blood from normal individual. Incubated anearobic 37°c 1-2 hrs. Treponemes adhere to erythrocytes in pressence of antibodies.
FTA (indirect IF)	Smears of killed T. palladium (nichol's strain) are prepared on slides and fixed. Patient is serum is allowed to react with smear+ fluorescien labelled antihuman immunoglobulin—apple green fluorescence positive.
FTA—ABS TEST	Patient serum is first absorbed with an extract of non—pathogenic treponeme (Reiter treponeme) to remove reagin. Smeared over the slide and over that fluorescein labelled antihuman immunoglobulin conjugate is added. In positive treponeme fluoresces.
TPHA	Sheep erythrocytes are sensitized with extract of T. palladium + patient's serum containing anti treponemal antibodies. Positive cases : clumps

Table 41: Serological test for syphillis

CHOICE OF SEROLOGICAL TEST	
Screening test	VDRL test and RPR test
Confirmatory test	TPHA and FTA—ABS test

Table 42: Positive predictive value of diagnostic test in syphilis diagnosis

Test	Primary stage	Secondary stage	Latent stage
VDRL	70%	100%	70%
FTA ABS	80%	100%	65%
TPHA	65%	100%	95%

10

IDENTIFICATION, MORPHOLOGY, STAINING, SPECIES VARIATION AND LABORATORY DIAGNOSIS OF FUNGI

S.No.	Topic
1.	Introduction
2.	Specimen Selection and Specimen Collection
3.	Specimen Transport, Storage And Processing
4.	Direct Microscopic Examination
5.	Culture Methods
	Sabouraud's Dextrose Agar (SDA):
	Cornmeal agar
	3. CHROM Agar
	4. Growth in Sabouraud's Dextrose Broth

6.	Physiological and Bio-chemical Characterization 1. Sugar Assimilation Test a. Auxanographic Technique b. Classical Wickerham method c. Automated Commercial System 2. Sugar Fermentation Test.
7.	Immune Diagnosis 1. Test for detection of Antibodies: 2. Tests for detection of Antigen to Candida species 3. Detection of Cell Mediated Immunity 4. Other Tests a. Detection of Fungal Metabolites. b. Molecular Biology Techniques

Identification, Morphology, Staining, Species Variation and Laboratory Diagnosis of Fungi

INTRODUCTION

Candida species are the most common opportunistic agents causing infections in humans. Their severity is greatly enhanced in the presence of predisposing factors such as immunosuppressive drug therapy, diabetes, prosthetic devices, etc. the clinical signs and symptoms and existence of predisposing factors will be helpful in determining the significance of the isolate. Hence, a valuable contribution can always be made by laboratory in establishing the diagnosis.

Specimen Selection and Specimen Collection:

Laboratory diagnosis of fungal diseases starts with careful

collection of appropriate clinical sample. The specimen must contain the viable etiological agent, if it is to be recorded and identified. The anatomic site in which the organism is present must be carefully selected and the specimen collected in such a manner that it will allow the fungus to remain viable in its natural state without contamination.

Glenn D. Roberts and Goodman criteria for specimen collection (2005)

1. Collect the specimen from an active lesion: old "burned out" lesions often do not contain viable organisms.
2. Collect the specimen under aseptic conditions.
3. Collect a sufficient amount of the specimen.
4. Collect specimens before instituting the therapy.
5. Use sterile collection devices and containers.
6. Label the specimens appropriately.
7. All clinical specimens should be considered as potential bio-hazards and should be handled with care, using universal precautions.

SPECIMEN TRANSPORT, STORAGE AND PROCESSING:

For the best results, all clinical specimens should be microscopically examined and cultured as soon as possible, except for blood and corneal scrapping which are cultured immediately. Specimens should not be frozen nor allowed to dry out.

when specimen reaches the laboratory they must be

appropriately processed to ensure viability of the etiological agent and to minimize the chances of contamination.

Direct Microscopic Examination:

Direct microscopy is a simple and economical approach for the detection of Candida species. However a negative result from microscopy should not be regarded as a definitive negative evidence for the presence of Candida species.

1. The preferred method for direct examination of clinical specimen is the wet mount technique using 10-40% KOH which helps in clearing the specimen of cells and debris.
2. It is also helpful to add Parker's ink or the Lacto Phenol Cotton Blue stain which enables easier demonstration of the fungal elements.
3. In addition to the above methods, fixed smears can be stained using Gram's or Giemsa stains. Tissue biopsies can be stained using Periodic Acid Schiff or Gomori's methanamine silver staining.
4. The most recent development involves use of Calcoflour white, a fluorochrome, with affinity for chitin and glucon which makes demonstration of fungal elements, possible with a fluorescent microscope.

Direct microscopic examination will reveal the presence of budding yeast cells or pseudohyphae. These cells and pseudohyphae commonly measure 3 to 5 μm diameter. These pseudohyphae show regular points of constriction, resembling lengths of sausages. These cells are strongly Gram positive. The microscopic examination serves only as an indication of candidiasis without defining the etiology, which can be established only by culture. Microbiological details of the various fungal pathogen in oral fungal disease are shown in table 47.

Culture Methods:

The isolation of Candida species from the respiratory, digestive or urinary tract is difficult to interpret as they exist as commensals. The isolation of candida species from naturally sterile environment like peritoneum, cerebrospinal fluid, joint aspirates, bone marrow etc should always be regarded as significant.

Culture methods in candida is shown in table 43

Table 43: culture methods of candida identification

Culture media:
1. Malt peptone Agar.
a. Malt peptone agar with antibiotics.
b. Malt peptone agar with antibiotics and Natamycin.
2. SDA media
a. SDA with Antibiotics.
b. SDA with Antibiotics and Cycloheximide.
c. SDA with Antibiotics and Natamycin.
d. SDA Broth

3.	Sugar Assimilation Test
4.	Potato dextrose Agar
5.	Corn meal Agar
6.	Christen's Urea Agar containing glucose
7.	Sugar Assimilation Test.

3. ***Sabouraud's Dextrose Agar* (SDA):**
   Glucose 20gm
   Peptone 10gm
   Agar 15gm
   Water 1 litre

Steam to dissolve and adjust to pH 5.4

1. A freshly collected specimen is spread on plates and incubated at 28°c Or / 37°c.
2. The colonies will be apparent with in 2-3 days.
3. Candida species appears as smooth, creamy, white and glistening colonies (Table 44)

Table 44: Culture character of candida by SDA

C. Albicans	Colonies are Creamy, smooth, white and glistering and older colonies are cream colored waxy or soft and smooth
C. Guillermondii	THIN, FLAT, glossy, cream to PINKISH colonies are seen.
C. Glabrata	Cream colored soft glossy smooth colonies. Cylindrical cells.

C. Krusei	Colonies are flat, DULL DIRTY, GREENISH YELLOW COLOR.
C. Parapsilosis	Colonies are YELLOWISH, glistering smooth.
C. Stellatoidea	Small creamy and smooth colonies (ON BLOOD AGAR—STELLATE COLONIES)
C. Tropicalis	Dull soft, and WRINKLED COLONIES.
C. Pseudotropicalis	Creamy, RETICULATE OR SMOOTH colonies.
C. Viswanathi	Cream colored and soft glistering colonies

Macroscopic morphology of candida species on routine isolation medium (SDA) is rather similar. Candida species appears on SDA as smooth, although fine differences between the species can be noted.

Candida albicans:

1. Macroscopically the colonies are creamy, smooth, white and glistening, and older colonies are cream-colored waxy or soft smooth or wrinkled and with or without mucelial fringes.
2. Microscopically globose, short, ovid (5-7µm). Sometimes, elongated small and larger cells are seen.

Candida guillermondii:

1. Macroscopically, thin, flat, glossy, cream to pinkish colonies are seen.

2. Microsopically, short, ovoid cells (2-5 x 3-7 μm) and small cylindrical cells are seen.

Candida glabrata:

1. Macroscopically cream colored soft glossy smooth colonies are seen.
2. Microscopically small, round yeast cells (2-5 x 3-7) and small cylindrical cells are seen.

Candida krusei:

1. Macroscopically young colonies are flat, dull and dirty. Older colonies are greenish yellow, dull, soft, smooth or wrinkled with a dense growth of mycelium around the colonies.
2. Microscopically cells are cylindrical and a few are ovoid cells. Sizes may vary considerably (3-5 x 6-20 μm). Some may vary very long.

Candida parapsilosis:

1. Macroscopically younger colonies are soft, smooth, white, and sometimes lacy. Older colonies are creamy, yellowish, glistening, smooth or wrinkled.
2. Microscopically cells are short ovoid to long ovoid (2.5-4 x 3.5-9 μm).

Candida stellatoidea:

1. Macroscopically, slow growing, small, creamy and smooth colonies are seen (on blood agar it forms small stellate colonies, hence the name).
2. Microscopically, short, ovoid or long cells (4-8 x 5-10 m) elongated or epiculated cells are sometimes seen.

Candida tropicalis:

1. Macroscopically, younger colonies are creamy white and smooth, but later, they turn into dull, soft, and wrinkled, often with overgrowth of tough mycelium.
2. Microscopically, globose, ovoid or short ovoid cells are seen.

Candida pseudotropicalis (C. kefyr):

1. Macroscopically, younger colonies are creamy, and smooth in appearance. Older colonies are creamy to yellowish, dull, soft, smooth or reticulate.
2. Microscopically, cells are short, ovoid with few elongated cells (2.5-5 x 5-10 μm) with abundant pseudomycelium. The cells are elongated, falling apart and lie parallel like "logs in a stream".

Candida viswanathii:

1. Macroscopically, younger colonies are cream colored,

soft and glistening. Older colonies are creamy, soft to membranous, wrinkled and semi-dull in appearance.

2. Microscopically, globose, ovoid to cylindrical (2.5-7 x 4-12 µm) cells are seen.

Cornmeal agar: (Cornmeal+ Agar+Water)

1. Differential media for identification of species of candida.
2. In the corn meal agar plate load the test specimen by making a well in it.
3. Place a cover slip over it incubate at 22°c for 48 hrs. and
4. Examine the plate under microscope.
5. Culture character of candida in cornmeal agar method

Table 45: Culture character of candida by corn meal agar method

C. Albicans	Mycelium and pseudomycelium are well formed
C. Guillermondii	WELL BRANCHED MYCELIUM and PSEUDO HYPHAE.
C. Glabrata	ABSENCE OF HYPHAE.
C. Krusei	TREE LIKE / crossed match stick like pattern of mycelium
C. Paraspisolis.	MULTIPLE MYCELIUM. Gives a appearance of PINE FOREST
C. Stellatoidea	TREE LIKE PATTERN and SHORT.
C. Pseudotropicalis	PSEUDOHYPHAE ARE PARALLEL.

| C. Viswanthi | Mycelium branches at 90°c. |

The commonly used differential medium for identification of the species of Candida is—Cornmeal Agar, supplemented with *Tween 80*. Subcultures are done on the cornmeal Agar plates from the primary SDA plate by *Dalmau technique*. The growth of Candida can be identified by the presence of pseudo-hyphae resulting from the pinching off process of Conidia and Blastoconidia. Both unstained and stained wet mounts can be used to demonstrate the morphologic features formed on Cornmeal Agar plates.

The different species of Candida can then be inferred by noting down the following features.

Candida albicans:

Mycelium and Pseudomycelium formed with masses of Blastoconidia at internodes. Terminal thick walled thallicconidia (Chlamydospores) are formed by most of the strains.

Candida guillermondii:

Well branched pseudo-hyphae, bearing clusters of blastospores are produced but true hyphae are absent.

Candida glabrata:

Characteristic feature of this species is the absence of hyphae or pseudo-hyphae.

Candida krusei:

Elongated cells arranged in *"tree-like"* or *"crossed matchstick"* pattern are seen. Blastoconidia are elongated and grow in verticellate branches from mycelium.

Candida parapsilosis:

Thin pseudo-mycelium with much branching and verticils of few ovoid to elongated blastoconidia are seen, giving an appearance of *"Pine forest"*. Thick pseudomycelium and giant cells are formed.

Candida stellatoidea:

Pseudomycelium is branched in tree-like pattern composed mainly of short cells irregular clusters of blastoconidia at internodes. Sometimes blastoconidia are in long chains. Chlamydospores are rarely produced.

Candida tropicalis:

Abundant pseudohyphae composed of elongated cells with much branching blastoconidia singly along mycelium, or in clusters are seen. True hyphae are also formed. Some strains also produce chlamydoconidia. These differ from those of Candida albicans in that they do not have a supporting cell and cessation of production of those conidia on subculture.

Candida pseudotropicalis: Pseudohyphae are abundant and the cells are elongated and lie parallel. Blastoconidia are not abundant, and when present, are elongated.

Candida viswanathii:

Long wavy mycelium with irregular branches at angles upto 90°, which are globose to ovoid blastoconidia in chains are seen, verticillately arranged.

CHROM Agar:

1. Novel differential culture for isolation.
2. A single colony is streaked on to chrom agar plates and incubated at 37°c with carbon dioxide in dark—48 hrs.
3. Culture character of candida in Chrom Agar media (Table 46)

Table 46: Culture character of Candida by Chrom Agar media

C. Albicans	Light green
C. Glabarata	Purple
C. Tropicalis	Blue with pink yellow
C. Parapsilosis	Cream colored
C. Krusei	Pink

An important development was Chrom Agar system by Odds and Bernaerts in 1994 which uses chromogenic substances. It is based on the reaction between specific enzymes of different species and chromogenic substrates which results in formation of colored colonies.

This is a novel differential culture medium for isolation and presumptive to identification of different species of Candida and has revealed mixtures of Candida species in many types of clinical samples more often than would have been expected. A single yeast colony was streaked on to the plates and incubated at 37°C with carbon-dioxide in the dark and the results read after 48 hours.

The species of Candida can be identified by different colored colonies which are as follows:

1. Candida albicans : Light Green
2. Candida glabrata : Purple
3. Candida tropicalis : Blue with Pink hallow
4. Candida parapsilosis : Cream colored
5. Candida krusei : Pink (Rough, Fuzzy spreading)
6. Candida dubliniensis : Dark Green

CHROM agar contains various substrates for enzymes of yeast species. It has been demonstrated that β n-acetyl galactosaminidase which was produced by Candida albicans, enables chromogenic substrates to be incorporated into the medium and the isolates of these species were seen as Green colored colonies.

Alternatively, certain other substrates like Bismuth salts (Nickerson's medium), triphenyl tetrazolium chloride and phosphomolybdate can be incorporated into the SDA for producing colored colonies for differentiation of species of candida.

Growth in Sabouraud's Dextrose Broth:

This serves as an important differentiating method for various species of Candida. If a Ring around the surface of the tube at the broth interface, it indicates Candida tropicalis. Similarly, a thick pellicle creeping along the sides indicates Candida krusei, while growth occurring at the bottom of the tube indicates other species of Candida.

Germ Tube Production (Reynolds-Braude Phenomenon):

This phenomenon was first described by Taschdjian, Burchall and Kozinn in 1960. The principle of this test is the ability of Candida albicans and its variants to produce germ tubes when incubated with various substances like, human or sheep serum, rabbit plasma, egg albumin, saliva, tissue culture medium, thioglycolate trypticase soya broth and various peptone medium at 37ºC for 2 hours. Germ tube is defined as a filamentous extension from a Yeast cell that is about half the width and 3-4 times the length of the mother cell (*Hand mirror forms*). The germ tube produced by Candida albicans has no constriction at the neck (True hyphal structure).

1. Germ tube: filamentous extension from a yeast cell (half the width and 3-4 times of length of mother cell) (true hyphae structure no constriction at neck.)

2. C. albicans and its variants when incubated with human or sheep serum / rabbit plasma/ egg albumin / saliva—37 °c for 2 hrs.

3. Produces germ tube

Physiological and Bio-chemical Characterization:

The genus Candida and its species can be characterized by the pattern of their use of specific carbohydrate and nitrogen substances. Candida species can use carbohydrate both oxidatively (assimilation) and anaerobically (fermentation). The yeast species possessing the ability to ferment a given carbohydrate also assimilates that substance, but not necessarily vice-versa. Thus, the biochemical identification of Candida species is based primarily on assimilation and fermentation tests.

1. *Sugar Assimilation Test*:

   The different techniques for assessing the assimilation patterns are:

   1. Candida can use CH both oxidatively (assimilation) and anaerobically (fermentation)
   2. A yeast species which can ferment the Carbohydrate can assimilate, but not vice versa.
   3. *Auxanographic* **technique:**
   4. Over Agar medium plate, on which paper discs impregnated with different CH are placed. The

growth ability of yeast around disc indicates the assimilate to carbohydrate.

a. *Auxanographic Technique* (Warren, Hazen and Howell): This Technique employs minimal media agar plates (yeast nitrogen base agar) on which, paper discs impregnated with different carbohydrates are placed. The growth ability of yeast around a specific disc is an indication of its ability to assimilate the carbohydrate. This method is simpler, quicker and used routinely.

b. *Classical Wickerham method*: This method was proposed by Wickerham and Bruten in 1948. This method assesses assimilation by determining the ability of a given yeast isolate to grow in a set of defined minimal liquid media supplemented with different carbohydrates.

c. *Automated Commercial System*:

1. API 20C system (Bio Merieux, Basingstke UK)
2. API ID 32C
3. VITEK (Bio Merieux, Vivek, Inc, Hazelwood, MD)
4. Minitek (Becton Dickinson microbiology system, Cokeysville, MD)
5. Uni-Yeast-Tek (Flow Laboratories, Woodcock, UK) these are commercial systems that are ready to use and some are automated.

2. **Sugar Fermentation Test:**

Liquid media—peptone water supplemented with carbohydrates and indiator to asses the pH.and inverted durham's tube to access the gas production

The classical test involves liquid media like Peptone water supplemented with different carbohydrates, an indicator to assess the pH changes to measure acid formation or production and an inverted Durham's tube to access the gas production. The color change in the tube containing the particular sugar indicates the ability of yeast to ferment that carbohydrate. There are several modifications for assessment of gas production, such as use of semisolid media or a wax plug on top of the liquid medium.

Immune Diagnosis:

The basis of Immunodiagnosis is the patient's response to candida, as expressed by the presence of antibodies or CMI or the presence of fungal antigens in the patient's body fluids. As a consequence, different types of assays are involved in immunodiagnosis.

1. **Test for detection of Antibodies:**

   The tests used to detect antibodies of Candida are—Agglutination of latex coated particle, immunodiffusion, immune electrophoretic test systems, radio immune assay and enzyme immune assay.

For the detection of antibodies diagnostic for a Candidal infection, various Candida structures have been tried as antigens: Cell wall mannan, glucan polysaccharides, mixed cytoplasmic antigen preparation and antigens expressed exclusively by the hyphal forms of Candida albicans.

The most promoting antigens have been—purified enolase as it is a protein expressed at high levels in Candida albicans cytosol, hsp90, and stress protein. False negative results are the major problem of these tests because of less sensitivity and non competent immune status of Candidal patients.

2. *Tests for detection of Antigen to Candida species* The various antigens detected by different systems are:

1. Detection of mannan using enzyme immune assays like Pastorer latex agglutination systems incorporating monoclonal antibodies and Candida antigen detection systems incorporating polyclonal antibodies.
2. Detection of Glycoprotein antigen using cand-tec latex agglutination test.
3. Detection of 47-49 KDa protein, apparently enolase using ELISA.

Antigens are detected generally in serum. However, they can also be found in other body fluids, including urine. The antigen detection tests are more significant for diagnosis because they detect active infection. But they are not sensitive enough and hence lead to false negative results. Another false negative result may come from cases where the infective agent is one of the rare Candida species, which are not recognized by the detecting reagents.

3. **Detection of Cell Mediated Immunity**:

These are valuable in assessing immune-competence of patients but not for the diagnosis of Candidiasis. The tests used for the detection of CMI are:

Invivo tests like skin test, to evaluate DTH to Candidal antigen.

Invitro tests like Lymphocyte transformation test.

4. **Other Tests**:

a. **Detection of Fungal Metabolites**:

D—Arabinitol is produced by most species of Candida except Candida krusei and Candida glabrata. In serum and urine it can be detected by gas liquid chromatography and by the Enzymatic fluorometric method. Serum arabinitol levels can be elevated in patients with renal insufficiency, Mannitol interference and steroid therapy. These tests, hence give false positive results. To overcome this problem, determination of serum arabinitol / creatinine ratio has been advised.

b. *Molecular Biology Techniques*:

Use of specific DNA probes like P 450, 14-lanosterol de methylase, parts of 18Sr RNA gene complex, chitin synthetase gene and mitochondrial DNA, has proved to be useful.

RNA profiling

Electrophoresis using different techniques like contour clamped homogenous electric field, OFAGE (Orthogonal Field Agarose Gel Electrophoresis) or FIGE (Field Invasion Gel Electrophoresis).

Restriction enzyme analysis.

DNA amplification techniques like Polymerase Chain Reaction (PCR).

Table 47: Microbiological detail of various fungal pathogens in oral fungal disease

DISEASE	PATHOGEN	LABORATORY	PROCEDURE
Histoplasmosis	Histoplasma capsulatum (Dimorphic Fungus)	2-4 µm yeast cell. SDA ot BHI with cyclohexmide and chloramphenicol inoculated 37°c White colony and finger like projections appears at 25°c	SDA with cycloheximide. Yeast phase: 37°c Mycelial form: 25°c Finger like projections.
Blastomycosis	Blastomyces Dermatitidis (Dimorphic fungus)	10% KOH Direct examination—thick walled yeast cell with broad based bud.	SDA medium: Mycelial form— 25°c and Yeast phase—37°c
Paracocidioidomyoosis	Paracoccidioides brasiliensis Dimorphic fungus	10% KOH Direct examination: numerous yeast cell	SDA medium Mycelial form— 25°c and yeast phase—37°c
Cocidioidomycosis	Coccidioides immitis Dimorphic fungus	SDA—inoculated 25°c for 3 weeks.	Septate hyphae fragment into arthrospores— Infective
Cryptococcosis	Cryptococcus neoformans	India ink or nigrosisn shows round budding yeast cells. and clear halo.	SDA—37°c smooth cream colored colonies.
Aspergillosis	Aspergillus fumigatus	KOH preparation— dichotomous branching. (at an angle of 45°c)	SDA 25°c : Cream velvetty colonies : black dichotomotus branching.

11

IDENTIFICATION AND LABORATORY DIAGNOSIS OF VIRUS

1. Viral culture
2. Polymerised chain reaction
3. Blot assay
4. Enzyme Linked Immunosorbent assay
5. Immunofluorescence
6. Laboratory diagnostic list for viral disease

1. Viral culture: Viral culture is a laboratory procedure in which samples will be placed with a cell type that the virus is being tested for its ability to cause infection. The results of the viral growth in culture are detected based on the presence of cytopathic effects, metabolic inhibition, hemadsorption, interference and transformation. Viruses are anobligate intracellular parasites that cannot be grown on any inanimate culture medium. There are three methods available for the cultivation of viruses. It includes inoculation into animals, embryonated eggs or tissue cultures.

a. **Animal Inoculation method of viral culture:** This method is earliest type of inoculation methods. The viruses causing human diseases were inoculated in the human volunteers, however due to the higher risk involved in the methodology, animal inoculation method is lease recommended. This method is used 1) when no other method is available and 2) when the virus is relatively harmless. In the experiment of isolation of the polio virus by Landsteiner, the animal inoculation methodology was employed on monkeys. However, use of monkeys in the animal inoculation had limited application due to their cost and risk to handlers.

Non human primates are also used in the animal inoculation methods. The mice are the most widely accepted and used in the animal virology studies. The experiments that are conducted on mice may be inoculated by several routes such as intracerebral, subcutaneous, intraperitoneal and intranasal. The viral growth in the inoculated animal can be detected by one of the following changes 1) visible lesions or manifestations, 2)morbid or diseased state and 3) death. The major disadvantage of the animal inoculation are the immunological activity in the host system, which may interfere with the viral growth and also animals often harbor latent viruses. This may be one of the potential bias in conducting experiments in the non human models. To summarize, animal inoculation methodology are used in the experiments in detecting pathogenesis, epidemiology, immune response, and carcinogenesis.

b. **Embryonated eggs method of viral culture:** This method was first used for the cultivation of viruses by Good pasture in 1931. The process of virus culture in embryonated egg depends on the type of the egg which is used. During this procedure, the egg should be sterile and the shell of the egg should be intact and healthy. This method offers several sites for the cultivation of virus. The different sites of viral inoculation in embryonated eggs are: 1) chorioallantotic membrane 2) amniotic cavity, 3) allantoic cavity, and 4) yolk sac. A hole will be drilled in the shell of the sterile and intact embryonated egg, and a sample with viral suspension is injected into the fluid part of the egg. The growth of virus will be indicated by 1) the embryo cell damage, 2) by the formation of typical pocks or lesions on the egg membrane or 3) the death of the embryo. The inoculation of chorioallantoic membrane produces visible lesions, called as pocks. The morphology of pock are different in different group of virus. Inoculation into the amniotic sac is primarily employed in the isolation of influenza viruses. The yolk inoculation methods are used in the viral cultivation of chlamydiae and ricketsiae organism. Duck eggs are bigger and may have a longer incubation period in comparison with hen's egg.

c. **Tissue Cultures:**
The first experimental tissue culture study was performed to maintain the vaccine virus in rabbit cornea. The tissue culture studies were initially employed to study the morphogenesis and wound healing. The major

challenge in the tissue culture was related to bacterial contamination. However, due to the advent of antibiotics, the challenges related to the bacterial contamination was substantially solved. The three most common types of tissue cultures are organ culture, explants culture and cell culture. The cell cultures replaced embryonated egg method, as the cell culture method was preferred type of growth medium for many virus types. The cell culture can be handled like bacterial culture, and thus it is considered to be more convenient method. However, the major challenges in cell culture methods are due to the requirement of skilled technicians with experience in working.

1. **Organ culture:** Organ culture is useful for isolation of certain virus type that is more specific to the organ type. Example: tracheal ring organ culture for isolation of corona virus. The organ culture allows maintaining the tissue bits for days and weeks and preserves the original architecture and function.

2. **Explant culture:** Explant culture is employed for isolation of cells from the minced tissue. The tissue that is harvested in this procedure is termed as explants. Example: Adenoid tissue explants cultures are employed in the isolation of adenoviruses.

3. **Cell cultures:** Cell culture is a compound process in which cells are grown in the artificial environment. The proteolytic enzymes such as

trypsin are used to isolate the cells from the tissues. Mechanical shaking also helps the tissue to dissociate into cells. After dissociation, cells are washed and suspended in a growth medium. The essential constituents for the growth such as vitamins, glucose, amino acids are added, to facilitate the growth of isolated cells. Based on the chromosomal character, tissue origin; cell cultures are further classified into three types, such as primary cell cultures, diploid and continuous cell cultures.

2. Polymerised chain reaction (PCR)

It is the molecular technique based on the principle of DNA polymerization reaction, during which a particular DNA sequence is amplified and made into multiple copies. PCR is an *in vitro* technique where it helps to amplify the DNA without restrictions on the form of DNA. The main components of PCR technique are primer, DNA template. The DNA template or cDNA (complimentary DNA) contains the region of the DNA fragment to be amplified. Primers are the agents that determine the "beginning" and "end" of the region to be amplified. The five steps in PCR technique are initiation, denaturation, annealing, elongation, and extension. The initiation step includes the heating the sample tissue at 96°C for five (5) minutes. The imitation steps facilitates in melting of DNA strands and primers. The denaturation step includes the heat treatment of sample at 96°C for thirty (30) seconds. Denaturation procedures help in lysis of the hydrogen bonds that are located in nucleic acids. The annealing step includes the heat treatment of sample at 68°C for thirty (30) seconds. The annealing step will help in formation of ionic bonds between primer and template, however these bonds are weaker. Continuation of annealing step will help in formation of much more stable bond between the single stranded primer and temple and helps in formation of double stranded DNA molecule. The polymerase enzyme that is used in the PCR technique will help in attaching and copying the template and eventually will help in formation of DNA copy. Elongation step is achieved by the treatment of the sample at 72°C for forty five (45) seconds. This technique helps in formation and lengthening of newly copied double stranded DNA. The DNA obtained from the extension will be transferred to the gel electrophoresis and continued for analysis and interpretation of the test results.

3. Western Blot analysis:

The western blot analysis is a molecular biological technique used to detect protein in a sample tissue. This method uses the gel electrophoresis to isolate the denatured proteins by molecular weight. The isolated proteins are transferred by the use of nitrocellulose membrane and finally detected by one of the analysis methods such as colorimetric method, chemiluminescence, radioactive detection, and fluorescence detection.

This method was originated from the laboratory of Geogre Stark at Stanford. The name western blot was coined by Neal Burnette after the southern blot analysis that is used to detect DNA material. The different blot analysis includes western, northern, and southern blot analysis. The Western blot analysis is a technique used to detect specific proteins in the sample.

Northern blot analysis is a technique used to detect RNA in the sample tissue. Southern blot analysis is used in detection of specific DNA sequence in the sample tissue.

The steps in western blot analysis are tissue preparation, gel electrophoresis, transfer, blocking, detection and analysis. The sample for this technique can be obtained either from tissue or cell culture. The tissue samples are subjected for mechanical breakdown by the use of homogenizer or by ultra-sonication. During the homogenization and tissue preparation phase, the enzymes such as protease and phosphatase inhibitors are often used to prevent the digestion of the sample by its own enzymes. The tissue preparation is done at lower temperature to avoid the protein denaturation and degradation. The proteins located in the sample tissue are isolated based on molecular weight with the use of gel electrophoresis. The gel electrophoresis is employed in the western blot analysis to facilitate the isolation of protein molecules based on the size, and shape. The isolated proteins are then transferred by the use of nitrocellulose membrane. This step allows the proteins to be accessible for antibody detection. To avoid non specific protein interaction between the protein and antibody, blocking step is employed. The blocking of non specific binding of proteins are achieved by the placement of membrane called Bovine Serum Albumin, or non fat dry milk. The detection of the protein is achieved by the antibody linked with enzyme, which provides colorimetric or photometric indication.

4. Enzyme Linked Immunosorbent assay:

Enzyme linked Immunosorbent assay (ELISA) is a immunological laboratory method that is employed to detect and quantify the specific antigen or antibodies in a tissue sample. The test uses antibodies and color change to identify the presence of antigen or antibody in a tissue sample. ELISA utilizes enzyme labeled antigens and antibodies to detect the biological molecule. The most frequently used enzyme in this method are alkaline phosphatase, and glucose oxidase. 96 well microtiter plates with antigenic fluid are used in the in the initial phase of the test. The antigen in the microtiter is allowed to bind to a specific antibody. After binding with the specific antibody, it is subsequently detected by a secondary enzyme coupled with antibody. A color substrate that is added in the method will help in the color change or fluorescence and indicates the positivity/ presence of antigen in the tissue sample. The enzyme linked secondary antibody reacts with color substrate and cause the breakdown of color substrate. The breakdown of color substrate will help in the visible color change.

5. Immunofluorescence:

Immunofluorescence is a molecular method of determining the location of antigen or antibody in a tissue section or smear by the pattern of fluorescence resulting when the specimen is exposed to the specific antibody or antigen labeled with a fluorochrome. The two major types of Immunofluorescence are direct and indirect technique. In the Direct technique, the antibody will be conjugated directly with the flurochrome and are used to detect the antigen in the tissue sample. Whereas, Indirect technique involves the interaction between the antigen and antibody in the serum sample.

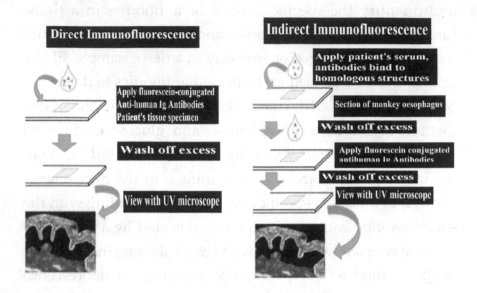

The tissue sample are recommended to store and transported in Michel's medium. Michel's medium contains ammounium sulphate, which will help in precipitating antibodies and other inflammatory proteins in the sample tissue. The second ingredient in the Michel's medium is enzyme inhibitor in citrate buffer with magnesium sulphate. The sample tissue can be placed in Michel's medium for the maximum of 24 to 48 hours. Normal saline can also as a transporting medium.

Direct Immunofluorescence:

To freeze the tissue specimen, the specimen should be immersed in liquid nitrogen and stored at 70°c. The procedures are conducted on less than 6μm cryostat sections of unfixed sample tissue. The sections are then washed with 0.1M phosphate buffered saline(PBS), with three changes for thirty minutes. The excess phosphate buffered saline is drained and wiped around section with cellulose tissue. The tissue section with diluted conjugate is allowed to react for thirty minutes at room temperature. The excess conjugate is allowed to drain with three changes of phosphate buffered saline solution for thirty minutes. The sections are mounted using 1,4 - Diazabicycoloctane (DABCO) solution. The edges of the cover slip are further sealed by polyvinyl alcohol/nail varnish. Upon completion of the latter step, the preparation can be viewed in fluorescent microscope. The slides should be stored at 4°c for longevity.

Indirect Immunofluorescence:

Indirect Immunofluorescence is a test in which patient serum is examined for the presence of antibodies to a defined antigen. Patient serum is diluted in phosphate buffered saline in 1:10 ratio. The suitable sections are selected and the serum dilution is exposed to the section for thirty minutes. The sections are usually taken from one of the tissues such as rat liver, kidney and thyroid tissue from human or monkey. The sections are then washed with phosphate buffered saline solution for 30 minutes with three changes. The excess phosphate buffered saline solution are removed by dabbing with cellulose tissue. The sections are further covered with diluted antihuman immunoglobulin/FITC conjugate. The excess conjugate is drained after thirty minutes and washed with phosphate buffered solution for another thirty minutes. Mount the tissue section as outlined in direct Immunofluorescence method. The section can be viewed under fluorescence microscope.

6. Laboratory diagnostic of viral infections:

It can be concluded that the detection of viral in infectious state can be detected and confirmed by one of the above mentioned methods. The laboratory diagnostic test of viral infections can be broadly categorized into growth detection by cell culture methods, detection of virus specific antibodies in the blood, detection of virus antigens, detection of viral genomic material, microscopic observation of virus particles by electronic microscopy, viral inclusions by cytology and histopathology techniques, or hemagglutination assay.

The laboratory investigation methods of certain oral infections are listed such as: herpetic stomatitis detection includes oral smear/exfoliative cytology and submit for papanicolaou test, direct immunofluorescence, ELISA or PCR technique. Herpese zoster infections can be detected by tzanck test, direct immunofluorescence ELISA or PCR technique. The Molluscum Contagiosum infection can be detected by papanicolaou test. The laboratory methods for Mumps are complement fixation test, hemagglutination method, ELISA, or Serum amylase levels. The laboratory methods for Epstein barr virus are Paul bunnell test, Indirect Immunofluorescence, or ELISA. The Human papilloma infections can be detected by Papanicolaou test, cytology, histopathology, ELISA or PCR. The HIV infections can be detected by ELISA, rapid assay, western blot test, or PCR technique. Three strategies for laboratory HIV infections were proposed. In strategy I, serum is tested with one ELISA or Rapid assay. Serum samples that are reactive are considered to be HIV antibody positive. Serum that is non reactive is considered to be a HIV antibody negative. In strategy II, sera reactive in ELISA or rapid assay of strategy I are retested using second ELISA or rapid assay. The ELISA or rapid assay are employed with different antigen preparation.

Serum samples that are reactive both test are are considered to be a HIV antibody positve. Where as serum that is non reactive is considered to be a HIV antibody negative. In strategy III, involves retesting the serum sample that were positive in two previous strategies. A third ELISA/rapid assay are conducted. The test interpretation can be drawn as sera reactive on all three strategy test are considered to be HIV antibody positive. Serum samples that are non reactive on strategy I, and II test are considered to be HIV antibody negative. Serum samples that are reactive in strategy I, II and non reactive in III test is considered to be equivocal.

12

ANTIBIOTIC SUSCEPTIBILITY TEST

Synoynms:

Culture sensitivity test
Antimicrobial susceptibility test
Pathogen please.

Definition: *"Evaluation of interactions between the isolated bacteria and Antimicrobial agent, needed invitro—and termed as Antimicrobial susceptibilty test."*

Purpose:

1. Whether an infectious agent is present.
2. Choice of Antimicrobial agent and its dose in therapy. (table 48)

Table 48 Choice of antibiotics:

S.No.	Species	Antibiotics
1.	Staphylococcus spp.	Gentamycin, tobramycin, amikacin, erythromycin, roxithromycin / azithromycin, clarithromycin, chloramphenicol, doxycycline, tetracycline, norfloxacin, lomefloxacin, levofloxacin, gatifloxacin, amoxicillin / ampicillin, cefazolin, cefpriome, clavulanic acid.
2.	Streptococcus Spp.	To be tested in Mueller hinton agar media with 5% sheep RBC Ampicillin, Pencillin, Erythromycin, Azithromycin, clarithromycin, co trimoxazole, cefotaxime, chloramphenicol, amox-clavulanic acid, cefepime, gatifloxacin, levofloxacin.

Antibiotic susceptibility test:

1. Disc diffusion 2. Dilution method

   a. The stoke's Method. a. Broth dilution method
   b. Modified Kirby—Bauer Method b. Agar diliution method

1. Disc diffusion method:

—For determine the drug susceptibility of the isolate there are two techniques.

- The difference between disc diffusion and dilution method are shown in table 51.

a. **The stoke's method:**

- Although in the past this method was the technique of choice but as this method has some limitations, so at present it has only a historical importance.

b. **Modified Kirby—bauer method:**

- On world wide scale the most popular method is the Kirby bauer method. It was subsequently modified and updated by the NCCLS (National Committee for Clinical Laboratory Standards now named as CLSI, USA.)

- The zone diameters that are generated by the test are meaningless without reference to the minimum inhibitory concentration (MIC) correlates and interpretative guidelines, published by the CLSI. (see Table NCCLS)

Preparation of culture plates: (Figure 14)

1. Preparation of plates.
2. Preparation of inoculums.
3. Inoculation of inoculums
4. Incubation
5. Interpretation
6. Results.

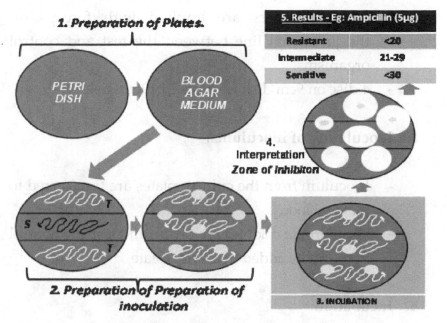

Figure 14 Schematic presentation of culture sensitivity test

1. **Preparation of plates:**

    - Medium allowed to cool to 50°c and add 5% blood agar.
    - Pour the medium in petri dishes to a depth of 4mm (25ml in a 9cm dish.)
    - Before inoculation dry the plate with lid agar so that there are no droplets of moisture on the agar surface.

2. **Preparation of inoculums:**

    - Take 2-3 similar type of colonies and incubate in nutrient broth an incubate 3-4 hrs at 35-37°c.
    - Transfer a loopful of control inoculums to 1/3 sides of pre dried medium plate.

- Antibiotic discs are applied with forceps on the junctional line between the test and control organisms.
- 4 disc on 9cm dish / 6 discs in 10cm dish.

3. Inoculation of inoculums:

- Inoculum from the culture plates are transferred to plate by loops.
- Well formed colonies are taken, and test and control both can be added in a same plate.

4. Incubation:

- Test and control is allowed are incubated overnight at 35°c-37°c.

5. Interpretation of plates:

- Interpretation is based on zone of inhibition around the disc and maximum zone in mm is noted. (table 50)
- Results are given as either "resistant" or "sensitive" strains of organisms.
- Factors influencing the zone of inhibition are shown in table 49.

Table 49: Factors that influence the zone of Inhibition

1.	DIFFUSIBILITY OF DRUG
2.	DISC CONCENTRATION
3.	NATURE and COMPOSITION OF MEDIUM
4.	MEDIUM THICKNESS
5.	PRESENCE OF INHIBITORY / STIMULATORY SUBSTANCES.
6.	Ph
7.	TIME OF INCUBATION

Eg: Ampicillin:

- Resistant : < 20mm
- Intermediate: 21-29
- Sensitive: <30mm

Table 50: Representing the disc and dilution method.

Drug	Disc Con	Inhibition Zone in mm.		
		Resistant	Intermediate	Sensitive
Ampicillin	10µg	<20	21-29	<30
Chloramphenicol	30µg	<12	13-17	<18
Erythromycin	15µg	<13	14-17	<18
Pencillin	10 units	<20	21-29	<30
Methicillin	5µg	<9	10-13	<14
Sulphonamides	300µg	<14	15-19	<20

Table 51: Disc diffusion and dilution test

Disc Diffusion Test		Dilution Test	
Stoke's Method	Kirby—Bauer Method	Broth Dilution Method	Agar Dilution Method
1. Not a technique of choice, due to limitations.	1. A suitable method for use in diagnostic laboraties, incorporate built in controls	1. Employed when therapeutic dose is to be regulated accurately in the treatment. 2. Too Laborious for routine use 3. When small degree of resistance to be demonstrated.	
1. Uses filter paper discs, 6.0mm in diameter	1. Uses the filter paper discs according to ICS by NCCLS— CLSI, USA. 2. Standard strains inoculated in middle third of plate. 3. Test strain inoculated in upper and lower third of plate 4. Antibiotic discs are applied between standard and test	1. Only one strain can be treated with one control. 2. Serial dilutions of drug in broth are taken in tubes. 3. MIC: lowest concentration of drug inhibits growth. 4. MBC: that kills the bacterium.	4. When several strains are to be tested at a same time. 5. Serial dilutions of drug in broth are taken in tubes. 6. MIC: Lowest concentration of drug inhibits growth. 7. MBC: that kills the bacterium.

Broth dilution method: (Table 52)

1.	Arrange 2 rows of 11 sterile capped tube in rack.
2.	In a sterile screw capped bottle—prepare 8 ml of broth, containing concentration of antibiotic required for first tube in each row. Then-> transfer 2ml broth to first tube in each row.
3.	Using sterile pippete, add 4 ml of broth to remaining 4ml in screw capped bottle Then—> transfer 2ml broth to second tube in each row.
4.	Continue preparing dilutions in this way to 10th tube.
5.	Antibiotic free broth to be placed in the last tube in each row.
6.	Inoculate 1 row with a drop of diluted overnight broth of TEST ORGANISM. and Similarly in 2nd row inoculate CONTROL SPECIES ORGANISM and Incubate all tubes at 37°c for 24 hrs.

13

ORGANIZATION OF THE CLINICAL LABORATORY

1. Function.
2. Staffing.
3. Management.
4. Elements of service.

   a. Guidance to users.
   b. Delivery of specimen.
   c. Request forms.
   d. Reception of specimen.
   e. Section of the laboratory.
   f. Choice of test.
   g. Reading of results.
   h. Wording of reports.
   i. Issue of reports.
   j. Computerization of reports.
   k. Laboratory manual.

5. Accomodation.

6. Safety precautions.

1. Function:

- Main work of clinical laboratory is to examine specimens from patients for the presence of potentially pathogenic microorganism.
- The purpose is quickly & economically to obtain information, that will help clinician to treatment patients.
- It is to serve the needs of clinical and preventive medicine, rather than advancement of microbiological science.
- Infection can progress very rapidly, so that speed of reporting is often more important than absolute certaininity of finding.
- In particular circumstances, however detailed identification of an infecting organism may be required as a guide to clinical management or an aid in helping epidemiological tracing.
- Principal problem of organizing a bacteriological service are

1. Determining the choice &
2. Sequence of test to be applied to each category of specimen.
3. Proper balance between economy of labor speed of reporting and precision of results.

- If there are sufficient resources, some applied research can be done on materials received in clinical laboratory and separately from routine diagnostic work.
- In addition to their maintenance of providing helpful reports on submitted specimens, the staff should take steps to inform all potential uses of services, the supply of specimen containers, the procedure of collecting specimen and arrangement for transportation of specimen.

2. Staffing:

- Staffing of clinical laboratory will vary with the kind and extend of clinical and preventive services it supports and the availability of finance of accomodiation.
- A population of about 2,50,000 will commonly receive about 1,50,000 specimen a year, it's staff may ideally include:

   a. 2 trained career grade graduates.

      i. 2 trained in Medicine & Microbiological sciences (consultant)
      ii. 1 Non—medically qualified scientist trained in microbiological research (top grade / principal grade scientist)

   b. 1 or 2 medical / science graduate in the training grade that lead to senior post.

    c.   Medical laboratory aids—cleaners.

    d.   4-5 clerical staff.

- **Medically qualified staff** have a special role in organizing the laboratory work in way best adopted to serve the needs of clinical and preventive medicine, in determing the kinds of examination to be made on particular specimen and deciding the content of reports.

- They are also qualified to give advice on:

1. Interpretation of results.
2. Problems of diagnosis.
3. Prevention and treatment.
4. Implication in advancement of medicine.

- **Research trained scientist:**

1. Special role in introducing and evaluating new tests & Procedures.
2. Establishing system of internal quality control.
3. Familiarity with current literature and
4. Habit of communication with other scientist and to appreciated the implication of advances in science of laboratory technology.

Techinical staff:

- Carry out most of the procedure at laboratory bench.
- Senior technical staff have a major responsibility for
    1. Day to day control of work on technical staff.

2. Recruitment, training & discipline of staff.

3. Maintenance of equipment, laboratory safely and

4. Ordering and control of supplies (stock management.)

- *As far as practicable, staff in the different categories should work side by side and learn as much as possible of each other's skill & knowledge.*

- Thus medically qualified staff should not confine themselves to reporting and advisory duties, but should become technically proficient in common bench procedures.

- This helps in full understanding of relevant scientific training and management issues.

> *Flexibility, co—operation and good will among the different categories of staff are essential for efficient performance of work in a clinical laboratory.*

3. Management:

- Appointment of director of laboratory / a management by laboratory committee represented by doctor.

- Director should be medically, scientifically / technically qualified.

- Director made responsible for

1. Standards of performance,

2. Expenditure,

3. Control of staff &

4. Strategy & organization of service.

- It's better to transfer the headship from time to time.
- Management by a committee may delay hence; director should make decision with out delay.
- He should determine his policies after wide and frequent consultation with senior members of categories of staff.

4. Element of the service:

a. Guidance to users.
b. Delivery of specimen.
c. Request forms.
d. Reception of sepecimen.
e. Section of laboratory.
f. Choice of test.
g. Reading of results
h. Wording of Reports.
i. Issue of reports.
j. Computerization of reports.
k. Laboratory manual.

a. Guidance to users:

- Should issue guidance to potential users of service in leaflet / booklet to

i. Hospital units.
ii. Medical staff.
iii. Family doctors.
iv. Environmental health officers.

- Leaflets should give

i. Address and telephone of laboratory.
ii. Range of examinations undertaken in laboratory.

iii. Describe the correct procedures for collecting each kind of specimen from patients.

iv. Safety precautions from likely to contain specially dangerous pathogens.

b. Delivery of specimens:

- Collection & delivery are usually done with in hospital in which the laboratory is located.
- Special van service from other hospitals, clinics and general practice health centres.
- Suitable boxes / trays should be provided for safe transport of specimen containers.
- Postal regulation specifying the types of containers and packing must be well made.

c. Request form:

- Designed in such a way as to require the clinician to give all the information they may be needed by laboratory staff. To determine the kind of examination to make on each specimen.
- Nature and source of specimen:
- Type of examination
- Patient name, age, sex, address, occupation and recent foreign travel.
- Hospital unit, signature, address and telephone number of requesting physician.
- Details of any current antibiotic therapy (to interpret the results of culture.)

- Request form must be submitted in duplicate, so that one copy can be used at bench and other for record purpose.

d. Reception of specimen:

- Should be done in separate room.
- Should be done by trained staff in appropriate safety precautions and procedure for dealing with leaking specimen.
- Recording of such specimen and information of same to patient.

    i. Name of the patient.
    ii. Place of collection of specimen.
    iii. Date of arrival of specimen.

- A laboratory serial No. is allotted to each specimen—(triplicate)

    i. Specimen container.
    ii. Request form.
    iii. Entry in reception book.

e. Sections of laboratory:

- If specimen received each day are numerous, divided in to 2 groups.

Ist Method:

- All specimen of all kinds received from a particular user group.
- **Eg:** clinic / hospital wards / general practice are allocated to a given group of sections.

Advantage:

- Continuous experience dealing all kinds of specimen helped to correlate the results for different kind of specimen received from same patient.

IInd Method:

- All specimen of particular kinds are allocated to sections specializing in examination of the kind of specimen.

- **Eg: 1.** Urine.

    2. Feaces,
    3. Pus / exudates / CSF,
    4. Serological, etc.

Advantage:

- Speed of working, accuracy and precision in field.
- However the range of experience would otherwise limited, hence staff should be from time to time be rotated among different sections.

f. Choice of tests:

- Laboratory should have carefully considered and clearly formulated policy for selection of stains, culture media, biochemical test, serological test & Antibiotics for sensitivity test to be used in examination of each kind of specimen.
- In most infections, the use of more than 2 or 3 methods of culture is recommended.
- Choice of test recognized by microbiological and he must given special attention.
- Selective approach avoids the waste of labor and materials used.

g. Reading of results:

- Available in stages on successive days.

- In significant cases, reports given preliminary to clinicians.

- For specimens such as respiratory tract, blood, infected exudates, the clinical significance of different organs need to be assessed in relation to clinical information given about the patient. It is preferred that reading of primary cultures and determination of reports should be done by senior staff.

- Microbiologist play a role in alert the serious clinical / epidemiological significances.

Eg: Presence of tubercle / typhoid bacilli.

h. Wording of Reports:

- That are understandable, instructive, relevant and reliable.

Eg: cultures yielded a profuse growth of enterobacter aerogenes, A saprophytic coli form bacillus that may be acting as an opportunistic pathogen in the patient.

- Not just interpretative comments, but also circumstances in which comments to be made.
- Finding of albus staphylococci in a blood culture to be reported with the content.
- Probably contaminant from skin and with out giving the antibiotic sensitivity.
- In compromised patient's:
  "possibly of clinical significance and antibiotic sensitivities are given.
- Acid fast bacilli—in specimen.
- AFB bacilli resembling tubercle bacilli seen in film culture for tubercle bacilli have been setup and will be reported later.
- **In case of negative reports,** "NO PATHOGENS WERE FORMED" imagine / means that search had been made for every kind of pathogen.

- **Eg:** if throat swab from acute sore that has been examined for S. pyogens.
- "Mixed throat organism present; Strep. Pyogens not found."
- "Viruses, mycoplasma and other pathogens not sought"

i. Issue of Reports:

- Scrutinized by senior medical staff before signature and issued.
- Copies of issual reports filed in laboratory.

j. Computerization of reports:

- Rapid, accurate operation of laboratory.
- Computerization of all details request form, entry, date and time of receiving specimen.
- Computer links the report to patient data from entry book.
- Laboratory statistics of pathogen, antibiotic sensitivities are also made.

k. Laboratory Manual:

- Sequence of examination to be made on each of different kind of specimen.
- Clear mention of methodology adopted of all tests with reference.

- Copies of relevant section should be reproduced in the manual for immediate references at bench.
- Manual should specify the selection of sequence of test to be applied to each different category of specimen.
- **Eg:** throat swabs from person over 4 years old suffering from acute sore throat for which he request is only "Pathogen Please" / Culture sensitivity.— means examined only for streptococcus pyogens and only be culture on aerobic and anerobic blood agar plates bearing bacitracin and pencillin disks for identification and sensitivity testing.
- Manual showed further state, the type of colonies and primary cultural plates.

5. Accomodation:

—As per Central Health Department and Public Health Laboratory Services.

—Requirement of laboratory safety must be taken in to account at early stage of design.

—Excluding circulation space, corridor, animal room, cloak room, toilets; about 1000m^2 of floor space would be required for population of about 2,50,000.

—Staff dealing with main section of bacteriological laboratory work accommodated in separate bays.

—At least 10m^2 of floor space should be available per person.

—2-3m of bench per technician and free wall space for floor standing equipment.

—A separate room with exhaust ventilated safety cabinets

required for work with dangerous pathogen like tubercle bacilli.

—Group of room required for

i. Sterilizing discarded specimens & cultures.

ii. clean containers & fresh cultures.

iii. Glass ware washing.

iv. For making & dispensing media.

- **Staff working** room must be separate from sterilizing and waiting room.
- A large Air conditioned room for storage of culture media, poured plates etc.,
- Separate rooms for chemicals and inflammable solvents.
- Small dark room for fluorescence microscopy.
- A large office with stationary, records required for clerical staff and computer cabinet.

6. Equipment:

i.   incubator,

ii. Refridgerator,

iii. Microscopes, ⎫⎬⎭ —*Main working room.*

iv. Water bath,

v.   Centrifuge.

vi. Rotary incubators & stands—*Separate room.*

vii. Autoclave.

viii. Culture media. ⎫⎬ Sterilizing room.

ix. Clean glass ware.

7. **Safety precautions:**

- Laboratory staff must be immunized against

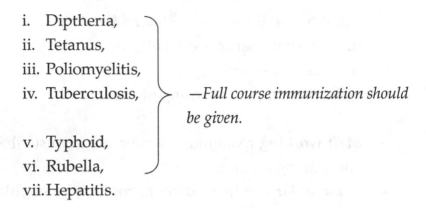

    i.   Diptheria,

    ii. Tetanus,

    iii. Poliomyelitis,

    iv. Tuberculosis,   —*Full course immunization should be given.*

    v.   Typhoid,

    vi. Rubella,

    vii.Hepatitis.

- Recognized prophylactic to

    i.   Anthrax

    ii. Plaque.

    iii. Clostridium botulism.

    iv. Rickettisae.

Safety cabinets:

- These cabinets provide a barrier between the worker and infectious material and are designed to prevent infection by splashing or by aerosol. According to united kingdom, three classes of cabinet are defined by British standard BS 5726: 1979.

Class I cabinets:

- Open fronted and rely on the walls, glass front and integral tray to contain spillage and splashes.
- An inward air flow provides a protection factor of at least 1.5×10^5
- The air is extracted from cabinet by a fan situated beyond the filter which ensures that no infective material is removed from the cabinet by the fan which itself cannot therefore be contaminated as long as the filter is intact.

Class II cabinets:

- Open fronted but have a flow of filtered air into the cabinet balanced by the extraction of air so that in theory the work in the cabinet is not contaminated by organisms in room air being sucked into the cabinet and the worker is not at risk of infection by organisms liberated from the cabinet.
- Although in ideal circumstances a class 2 cabinet can provide a protection factor equivalent to a class I, it is much easier for this protection to be reduced by mechanical or operational factors.

Class III cabinets:

- Totally enclosed, gloves for the worker being attached to the sealed front of the cabinet.
- They are scavenged by air entering and leaving the cabinet through HEPA filters, the circulation being such

that the air pressure in the cabinets is below that in the room. Sycg cabinets provide a high degree of worker protection and are the only ones permissible when dealing with category 4 pathogens.

- Plastic tents with filtered air inlets and exhausts ('flexible film isolators') are an attractive alternative to rigid class 3 cabinets.

- Theyare development of the tents designed by Trexler & Reynolds (1957) to hold gnotobiotic ('germ free ') animals and later adapted for the nursing of patients infected with a category 4 pathogen.

- Guidance on their used, testing and maintainence has been issued by the Advisory committee on Dangerous pathogens (1985).

- They may well play an increasing role in laboratories where work with dangerous pathogens is carried out.

Use of Class I and II cabinets

- These open—fronted cabinets must be sited carefully and should not be used if persons are moving about in the laboratory as draughts from doors, windows or those created by persons walking past a cabinet can draw particles eddying in the front of the cabinet back into the room.

- Care must be taken that the air from safety cabinet is discharged safely to the outside but never near ventilation intakes or open windows.

- Because these cabinets protect by virtue of a correct air

flow this must be checked daily by viewing the air flow indicator (Class I) and monthly with an anemometer.

- Good guidance on safety cabinets is presented and Howie code as well as detailed information by Collins (1983).
- It must be stressed that open fronted safety cabinets depend on air flow patterns for worker protection and cannot contain gross splashes or particles ejected from centrifuges, which must never be place in such cabinets.
- Similarly, air flow patterns can be disturbed by any obstruction and open fronted saftety cabinets, in particular must not be cluttered up with equipment.
- Untidy, overcrowded working condtions are not compatible with safety.
- Cabinets must be disinfected after working with pathogens and always before any maintenance or change of filter.
- At the end of a working day, wipe the inside walls and floor with a disinfectant. At the end of a cycle of work and in any case at weekly intervals, vaporize formalin inside the cabinet while the aperture of class 1 and 2 cabinets is occluded by a night door.
- The amount of formalin, 0.05 g/ m³ (approximately25 ml of formalin BP In a class I cabinet) is specified preferably vaporize it with a thermostatically controlled electric heater.
- Allow the vapor to act over night before purging by ventilation through the filter. UV lights are not recommended for the disinfection of safety cabinets.

FLOW CHART - I

Differentiation of gram positive coccus by CATALASE TEST

Gm positive coccus

CATALASE TEST

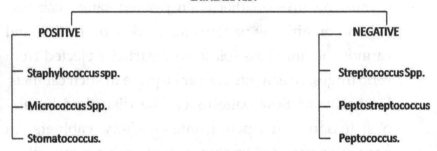

POSITIVE	NEGATIVE
Staphylococcus spp.	Streptococcus Spp.
Micrococcus Spp.	Peptostreptococcus
Stomatococcus.	Peptococcus.

FLOW CHART - II

Species identification of catalase positive gram positive cocci
Catalase positive gram positive cocci

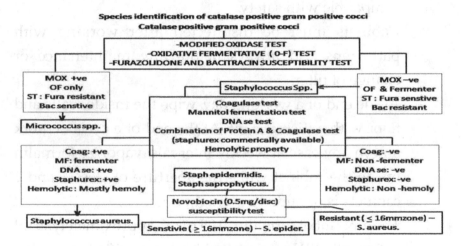

FLOW CHART - III

Species identification of catalase negative gram positive coccii

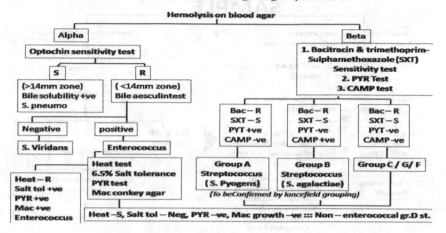

FLOW CHART - IV

LACTOBACILLUS

SALIVA

LB count count for DC

1. Mix Pt's saliva +10cc Sterile saline.

2. Make serial dilution of Saliva

3. Prep with Sterile N broth.

4. Distribute 0.1ml of different dilutions in
Different kulp's tomato peptone agar plates

5. Incubate the plates under microerophillic
Condition at 37°c for 3-4 days.

Count the colonies

More than 10^5 LB / ml of saliva is indicative of caries activity

FLOW CHART - V

ACTINOMYCES

SAMPLE

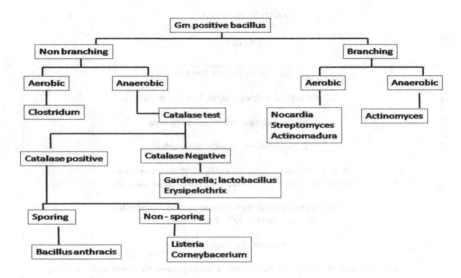

If visible granules are present (large firm round yellow color) pus

⬇

Wash & separate by adding with distill water & shaked

⬇

Granules are crushed in few drops of water, taken on 3 slides.

One is added 1- 2 drops of 20% KOH

⬇

Thin branching Threads .

2ⁿᵈ & 3ʳᵈ Allow to dry & fix with methanol for 1-2 mts.

⬇

Gm staining: Gm +ve branches & club Gm negative. ZN staining : Non AF Branching & Clubs Acid fast.

Inoculate in blood agar

⬇

Incubate at 37°c for 5-7 days

⬇

Colonies

Gm & AF staining

Catalase -ve

Inoculate in sucrose, glucose, lactose, maltose (fermented)

⬇

Actinomyces israllei

FLOW CHART - VI

Gm positive bacillus

Non branching

Branching

Aerobic

Anaerobic

Aerobic

Anaerobic

Clostridum

Catalase test

Nocardia Streptomyces Actinomadura

Actinomyces

Catalase positive

Catalase Negative

Gardenella; lactobacillus Erysipelothrix

Sporing

Non - sporing

Bacillus anthracis

Listeria Corneybacerium

168

FLOW CHART - VII

MYCOBACTERIUM TUBERCULI

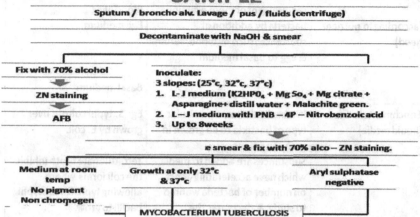

SAMPLE

Sputum / broncho alv. Lavage / pus / fluids (centrifuge)

Decontaminate with NaOH & smear

Fix with 70% alcohol

ZN staining

AFB

Inoculate:
3 slopes: (25°c, 32°c, 37°c)
1. L- J medium (K2HPO₄ + Mg So₄ + Mg citrate + Asparagine+ distill water + Malachite green.
2. L—J medium with PNB – 4P – Nitrobenzoic acid
3. Up to 8weeks

e smear & fix with 70% alco— ZN staining.

Medium at room temp
No pigment
Non chromogen

Growth at only 32°c & 37°c

Aryl sulphatase negative

MYCOBACTERIUM TUBERCULOSIS

FLOW CHART – VIII

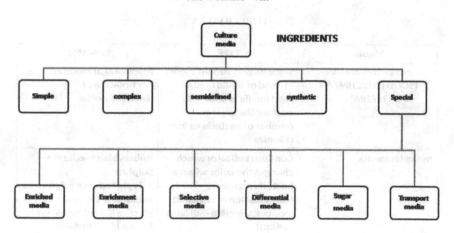

Culture media   **INGREDIENTS**

Simple | complex | semidefined | synthetic | Special

Enriched media | Enrichment media | Selective media | Differential media | Sugar media | Transport media

FLOW CHART – IX

MEDIA	TYPE	EXAMPLE
Enriched media (according to nutrient need)	Prepared to meet the nutritional requirement of more exacting bacteria by addition of substances such as blood, serum & egg to basal medium	Chocolate agar, Blood agar, Egg medium + Basal medium
Enrichment media (liquid media)	In mixed cultures, a particular type of bacteria to be grown in such conditions, - Substances are added to media, which have accelerating effect on number of bacteria wanted to study. & decreases the unwanted bacteria growth.	Eg: S. typhi culture over grown by E. coli. Tetrathionate broth inhibits the coli forms where allowing typhi & Paratyphi bacilli to grow.

FLOW CHART – X

Media	TYPE	EXAMPLE
SELECTIVE MEDIA (SOLID ENRICHMENT MEDIA)	Same as enrichment media Instead of liquid media – solid media is used – it enables the greater number of bacteria to form colonies	Manitol agar medium For isolation of staphylococcus.
Indicator media	Contains indicator which changes the color when a bacteria is grown . (combination of enriched media + selective indicator system)	Wilson blair medium + Sulphite s. Typhi reduces sulphite to sulphide in presence of glucose & contains S. typhi have a black metallic stream.
Sugar media	Contains fermentable substances along with indicator	Sugar + Hisserium for pneumococci.

FLOW CHART – XI

MEDIA	TYPE	EXAMPLE
Transport media	Used for delicate organisms, that may not survive during transport— gonococci, due to over grown by non pathogens— cholera, dysentry pathogens	Stuart medium Non— nutrient agar medium + reducing agent to prevent oxidation
TRANSPORT MEDIA	PIKE's media Streptococcus, Pneumococcus, H. influenza.	Blood agar + Crystal violet 1 in 10 lac & Sodium azide 1 in 16,000.
Anaerobic medium	For growing anerobes in air & preservation of anaerobic environment in culture	Robertson— bullock heart meat medium.
Differential media	Contains substances that bring out differing characterstics of bacteria & thus distinguishiable between them.	Mac— Conkey's media: Lactose fermenters — pink colonies Non— Lactose fermenters — Colorless.

FLOW CHART – XII

Laboratory diagnosis of syphillis

Demonstration of treponemes	1. Dark ground microscopy. 2. Direct fluorescent antibody staining for T. Pallidum (DFA – TP) 3. Treponemes in tissue. 1. silver impregnation method. 2. Immunofluorescent staining.
Serological test 1. Non treponemal test	1. VDRL 2. RPR 3. Kahn test & 4. Wasserman test
2. Treponemeal test	1. FTA , FTA – ABS test (Killed T. palladium) 2. TPHA (T.palladium extract) 3. TPI (uses Live T. palladium)

1. Cardiolipin antigen is an alcoholic extract of beef heart tissue to which lecithin & cholestrol is added – VDRL antigen

2. Non – specific antibody appears in blood of syphillitic patient – *"Reagin"*

DFA – TP	Smear of material to be test is made on glass side + Flourescent labelled monoclonal antibody Stained : appears, distinct sharply outlined apple green fluorescence.
VDRL TEST	Slide flocculation test : VDRL ANTIGEN + Reagin – visible clumps : positive
RPR Rapid Plasma Reagin	VDRL antigen suspended in choline chloride mixed with finely divided carbon particles. + patient serum / plasma Clumps : positive

Cardiolipin is non specific antigen may react with sera of patients who may not have syphillis, accounts for BIOLOGICAL FALSE POSITIVE REACTIONS (BFP)
Leprosy
Malaria
Relapsing fever
Hepatitis
SLE

FLOW CHART – XV

TP Immobilisation test (live T. Palladium	Test serum + actively motile Nichol's strain of T. pallidum & incubated anerobically. If antibodies are present the treponema are immobilised when examined under microscope.
Using killed T. palladium 1. TPA	Suspension of T. palladium is inactivated by formalin. This is mixed with test serum & Examined under dark ground microscopy. Treponema agglutinated in presence of antibodies.
2. TPIA	Suspension of inactivated T. palladium is mixed with test serum + complement + Fresh heparinized whole blood from normal individual. Incubated anaerobic 37°c 1-2 hrs. Treponemes adhere to erythrocytes in presence of antibodies.
FTA (indirect IF)	Smears of killed T. palladium (nichol's strain) are prepared on slides and fixed. Patient is serum is allowed to react with smear+ fluorescien labelled antihuman immunoglobulin – apple green fluorescence positive.

FLOW CHART – XVI

FTA – ABS TEST	Patient serum is first absorbed with an extract of non – pathogenic treponeme (Relter treponeme) to remove reagin. Smeared over the slide & over that fluorescein labelled antihuman immunoglobulin conjugate is added. In positive treponeme fluoresces.
TPHA	Sheep erythrocytes are sensitized with extract of T. palladium + patient's serum containing anti treponemal antibodies. Positive cases : clumps

CHOICE OF SEROLOGICAL TEST

Screening test	VDRL test & RPR test
Confirmatory test	TPHA & FTA – ABS test

Test	Primary stage	Secondary stage	Latent stage
VDRL	70%	100%	70%
FTA ABS	80%	100%	65%
TPHA	65%	100%	95%

FLOW CHART – XVII

Culture media for fungi:
1. Malt peptone Agar. a. Malt peptone agar with antibiotics. b. Malt peptone agar with antibiotics & Natamycin.
2. SDA media a. SDA with Antibiotics. b. SDA with Antibiotics & Cycloheximide. c. SDA with Antibiotics & Natamycin. d. SDA Broth
3. Sugar Assimilation Test
4. Potato dextrose Agar
5. Corn meal Agar
6. Christen's Urea Agar containing glucose
7. Sugar Assimilation Test.

FLOW CHART – XVIII

Culture technique for candidia

SDA:

Glucose 20gm Peptone 10gm Agar 15gm Water 1 litre Steam to dissolve & adjust to pH 5.4

A freshly collected specimen is spread on plates and incubated at 28°c
Or / 37°c.
The colonies will be apparent with in 2-3 days.
Candida species appears as smooth, creamy, white and glistening colonies

SDA

C. Albicans	Colonies are Creamy, smooth, white and glistering and older colonies are cream colored waxy or soft & smooth
C. Guillermondii	THIN, FLAT, glossy, cream to PINKISH colonies are seen.
C. Glabrata	Cream colored soft glossy smooth colonies. Cylindrical cells.
C. Krusei	Colonies are flat, DULL DIRTY, GREENISH YELLOW COLOR.
C. Parapsilosis	Colonies are YELLOWISH, glistering smooth.
C. Stellatoidea	Small creamy & smooth colonies (ON BLOOD AGAR – STELLATE COLONIES)
C. Tropicalis	Dull soft, & WRINKLED COLONIES.
C. Pseudotropicalis	Creamy, RETICULATE OR SMOOTH colonies.
C. Viswanathi	Cream colored & soft glistering colonies

FLOW CHART – XX

Corn meal Agar
(Cornmeal+ Agar+Water)

- Differential media for identification of species of candida.
- In the corn meal agar plate load the test specimen by making a well in it.
- Place a cover slip over it incubate at 22°c for 48 hrs. &
- Examine the plate under microscope.

FLOW CHART – XXI

Cornmeal agar media

C. Albicans	Mycelium & pseudomycelium are well formed
C. Guillermondii	WELL BRANCHED MYCELIUM & PSEUDO HYPHAE.
C. Glabrata	ABSENCE OF HYPHAE.
C. Krusei	TREE LIKE / crossed match stick like pattern of mycelium
C. Paraspisolis.	MULTIPLE MYCELIUM. Gives a appearance of PINE FOREST
C. . Stellatoidea	TREE LIKE PATTERN & SHORT.
C. Pseudotropicalis	PSEUDOHYPHAE ARE PARALLEL.
C. Viswanthi	Mycelium branches at 90°c.

FLOW CHART – XXII

DIAGNOSTIC APPROACH FOR VARIOUS FUNGAL

DISEASE	PATHOGEN	LABORATORY	PROCEDURE
Histoplasmosis	Histoplasma capsulatum (Dimorphic Fungus)	2 – 4 µm yeast cell. SDA ot BHI with cyclohexmide & chloramphenicol inoculated 37°c White colony & finger like projections appears at 25°c	SDA with cycloheximide. Yeast phase: 37°c Mycelial form: 25°c Finger like projections.
Blastomycosis	Blastomyces Dermatitidis (Dimorphic fungus)	10% KOH Direct examination – thick walled YEAST CELL WITH BROAD BASED BUD.	SDA medium: Mycelial form - 25°c & Yeast phase - 37°c
Paracocidioidomyoosis	Paracoccidioides brasiliensis Dimorphic fungus	10% KOH Direct examination: NUMEROUS YEAST CELL	SDA medium Mycelial form - 25°c & yeast phase - 37°c

FLOW CHART – XXIII

DISEASE	PATHOGEN	LABORATORY	PROCEDURE
Cocidioidomycosis	Coccidioides immitis Dimorphic fungus	SDA – inoculated 25°c for 3 weeks.	Septate hyphae fragment into arthrospores - Infective
Cryptococcosis	Cryptococcus neoformans	India ink or nigrosisn shows round budding yeast cells. & clear halo.	SDA - 37°c smooth cream colored colonies.
Aspergillosis	Aspergillus fumigatus	KOH preparation – dichotomous branching. (at an angle of 45°c)	SDA 25°c : Cream velvetty colonies: black dichotomotus branching.

FLOW CHART – XXIV

MUMPS

Diagnostic test
Complement fixation test
Hemagglutination method.
ELISA
Serum amylase levels.

PAPILLOMA

PCR

HIV

Immunological test	Specific test
1. Leucopenia & lymphopenia– 2000/mm³	1. Ag detection p24 – ELISA.
2. CD+T cell : < 200 /mm3. T4: T8 cell ratio reversed.	2. PCR
3. Thrombocytopenia	3. Western Blot test
4.Raised IgG & IgA levels	

EBV – INFECTIOUS MONONUCLEOSIS

White cell count	Leucocytosis & Relative lymphocytosis.
Serological test	Paul – Bunnell test
Immunoglobulin test	Indirect Immunofluoroscence.
Molecular test	ELISA.

HERPETIC STOMATITIS

Primary	Secondary
Smear – pap stain PCR technique.	Direct immunofluorescent ELISA

HERPES ZOSTER

Primary	Secondary
Tzanck test	Direct immunofluorescent

MOLLUSCUM CONTAGIOSUM

Diagnostic test
PAP Stain

FLOW CHART – XXVII

ELISA - HIV

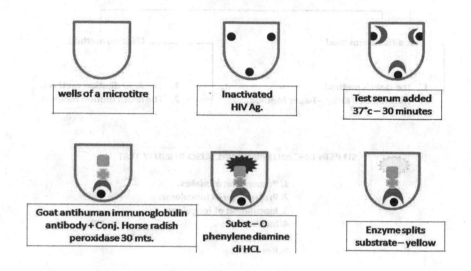

| wells of a microtitre | Inactivated HIV Ag. | Test serum added 37°c – 30 minutes |

| Goat antihuman immunoglobulin antibody + Conj. Horse radish peroxidase 30 mts. | Subst – O phenylene diamine di HCL | Enzyme splits substrate – yellow |

FLOW CHART – XXVIII

IMMUNOFLUORESCENCE

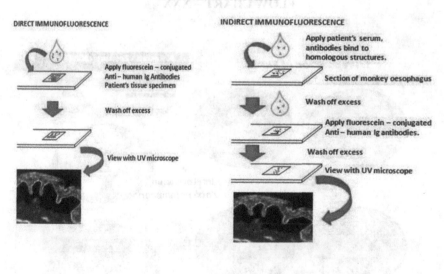

DIRECT IMMUNOFLUORESCENCE

Apply fluorescein – conjugated Anti – human Ig Antibodies Patient's tissue specimen

Wash off excess

View with UV microscope

INDIRECT IMMUNOFLUORESCENCE

Apply patient's serum, antibodies bind to homologous structures.

Section of monkey oesophagus

Wash off excess

Apply fluorescein – conjugated Anti – human Ig antibodies.

Wash off excess

View with UV microscope

FLOW CHART – XXIX

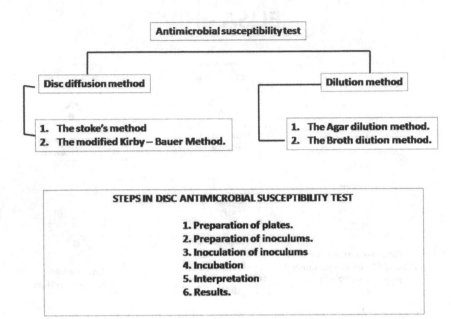

Antimicrobial susceptibility test

Disc diffusion method

1. The stoke's method
2. The modified Kirby – Bauer Method.

Dilution method

1. The Agar dilution method.
2. The Broth diution method.

STEPS IN DISC ANTIMICROBIAL SUSCEPTIBILITY TEST

1. Preparation of plates.
2. Preparation of inoculums.
3. Inoculation of inoculums
4. Incubation
5. Interpretation
6. Results.

FLOW CHART – XXX

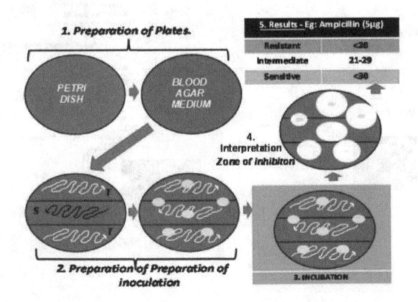

Printed in the United States
By Bookmasters